COPYCAT RECIPES

MAKING THE MOST POPULAR KETO RECIPES AT HOME - FAMOUS RESTAURANT COPYCAT COOKBOOK

NÚRIA OLAN

Copyright © 2021 NÚRIA OLAN

All rights reserved

Copyright © 2021 by NÚRIA OLAN. All rights reserved. No part of this book may be reproduced or transmitted in any form or by any means, electronic or mechanical, including photocopying, recording or by information storage and retrieval system, without the written permission of the author.

Editing by NÚRIA OLAN

- BREAKFAST RECIPES ---7
- COCONUT BARS ---8
- BLUEBERRY PANCAKE BITES ---10
- BREAKFAST BOWL ---12
- LOW-CARB CHEESECAKE ---13
- EGGS AND SAUSAGES ---15
- ALMOND FLOUR KETO PANCAKES ---18
- RANCH CAULIFLOWER CRACKERS ---19
- SCRAMBLED EGGS ---21
- FRITTATA ---22
- SMOKED SALMON BREAKFAST ---23
- BREAKFAST EGGS ---24
- EGGS BAKED IN AVOCADOS ---25
- BACON BREAKFAST AND SHRIMP ---27
- BREAKFAST PIE ---28
- MEXICAN BREAKFAST ---29
- BREAKFAST STIR FRY ---30
- BREAKFAST CASSEROLE ---31
- BREAKFAST SKILLET ---32
- BREAKFAST DISH ---33
- BREAKFAST PATTIES ---34
- SAUSAGE QUICHE ---36
- CAULIFLOWER BREAKFAST AND CHORIZO ---37
- BREAKFAST PORRIDGE ---38
- ITALIAN SPAGHETTI CASSEROLE ---39
- GRANOLA ---40
- BREAKFAST BOWL ---41
- ALMOND CEREAL ---42

BREAKFAST BREAD	43
BREAKFAST MUFFINS	44
CHICKEN BREAKFAST MUFFINS	45
BREAKFAST SANDWICH	46
AVOCADO MUFFINS	47
HERBED BISCUITS	49
BACON AND LEMON BREAKFAST MUFFINS	50
TURKEY BREAKFAST	52
BREAKFAST HASH	53
COCOA CEREAL NIBS BREAKFAST	55
CHIA PUDDING BREAKFAST	56
EASY CEREAL BREAKFAST	57
SWEET PANCAKES	58
PUMPKIN PANCAKES	60
DELICIOUS WAFFLES	61
THE PERFECT SMOOTHIE	62
BREAKFAST SMOOTHIE	63
CHICKEN QUICHE	65
CHICKEN OMELET	66
EASY SMOOTHIE BOWL	67
BREAKFAST TUNA SALAD	69
KETOGENIC RECIPES FOR LUNCH	72
CAESAR SALAD	73
PIZZA	74
CHOCOLATE PROTEIN PANCAKES	75
PIZZA ROLLS	77
STUFFED PEPPERS	78
BURGERS	79

AVOCADO EGG BAKE	80
ZUCCHINI DISH	82
TURKEY-PEPPER MIX	83
INGREDIENT ZUCCHINI LASAGNA	85
COLD AVOCADO AND CRAB SOUP	89
BALSAMIC CHICKEN	91
STEAK SALAD	93
SPINACH AND RED PEPPER FRITTATA	94
STUFFED AVOCADO	96
CHICKEN PAN WITH VEGGIES AND PESTO	97
CRAB CAKES	99
FRITTATA	100
PORK PIE	102
PATE	104
ZUCCHINI CRUSTED PIZZA	105
NOODLES SOUP	107
ROASTED CAULIFLOWER AND TAHINI YOGURT SAUCE	108
SPICY TUNA KEBAB	110
ASPARAGUS PRIES	112
GARLICKY GREEN BEANS	114
CREAMY CHICKEN POT PIE SOUP	116

Breakfast Recipes

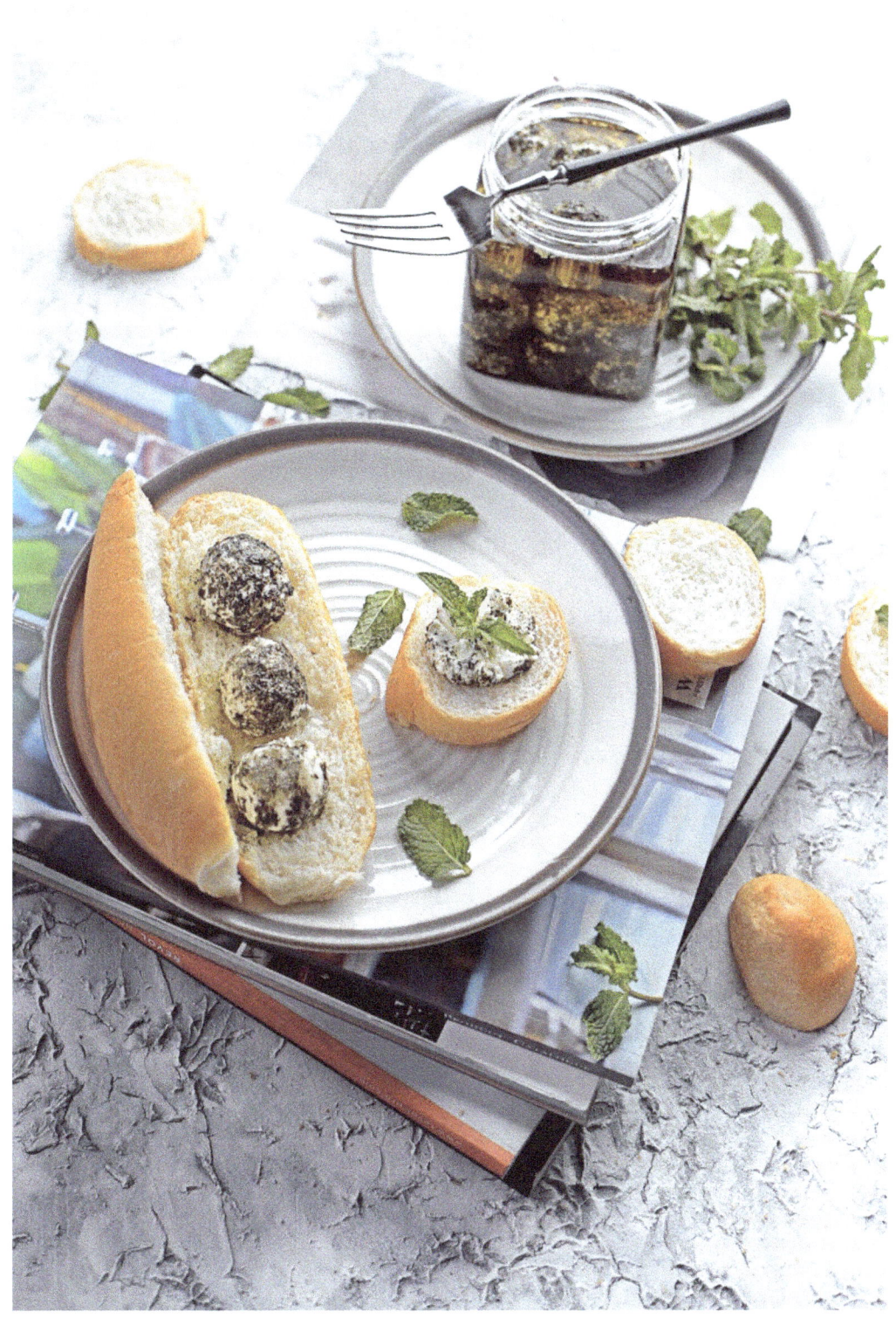

Coconut Bars

Preparation Time: 10 minutes **Cooking Time:** 0 minute **Servings:** 20

Ingredients:
- 3 cups of unsweetened shredded coconut
- 1 cup of coconut oil
- ¼ cup of liquid sweetener of choice

Kitchen Equipment:
- pan
- parchment paper

Directions:

1. Line a pan with a layer of parchment paper.
2. Combine the ingredients to make a thick batter.
3. Pour into the pan and freeze until firm.
4. Cut into squares and store until you want a delicious snack.

Nutrition: **Protein Counts:** 2g **Total Fats:** 11g **Calories:** 108

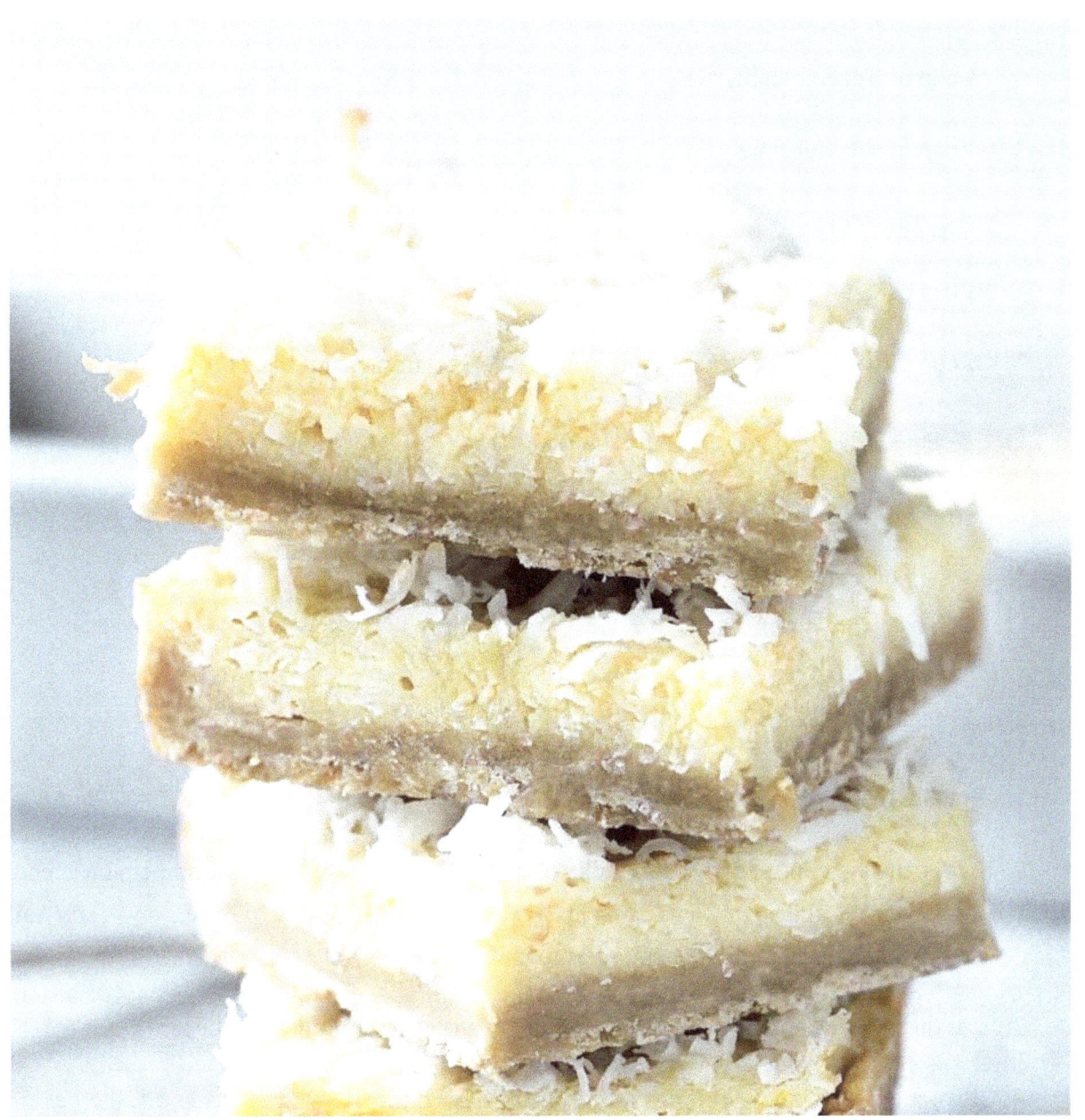

Blueberry Pancake Bites

Preparation Time: 10 minutes **Cooking Time:** 25 minutes **Servings:** 24

Ingredients:

- ½ cup of frozen blueberries
- ½ cup of coconut flour
- 1 tsp. of baking powder
- ½ tsp. of salt
- ¼ cup of swerve Sweetener
- ¼ tsp. of cinnamon
- ½ tsp. of vanilla extract, unsweetened
- ¼ cup of butter, grass-fed, unsalted, melted
- 4 Eggs, pastured
- 1/3 cup of water

Kitchen Equipment:

- oven
- immersion blender
- silicon mini muffin tray
- freezer bag

Directions:

1. Prepare oven at 350 degrees.

2. Crack the eggs in a bowl, add vanilla and sweetener, whisk using an immersion blender until blended and then blend in salt, cinnamon, butter, baking powder, and flour until incorporated and smooth batter comes together.

3. Let the batter rest until thickened and then blend in water until combined.

4. Take a 25-cups silicone mini-muffin tray, grease the cups with avocado oil, then evenly scoop the prepared batter in them and top with few blueberries, pressing the berries gently into the batter.

5. Situate the muffin tray into the oven and bake the muffins for 25 minutes or until thoroughly cooked and the top is nicely golden brown.

6. When done, take out muffins from the tray and cool them on the wire rack.

7. Place muffins in a large freezer bag or evenly divide them in packets and store them in the refrigerator for four days.

8. When ready to serve, microwave the muffins for 45 seconds to 1 minute or until thoroughly heated.

Nutrition: Calories: 188 **Fat:** 13.8g **Protein:** 5.7g

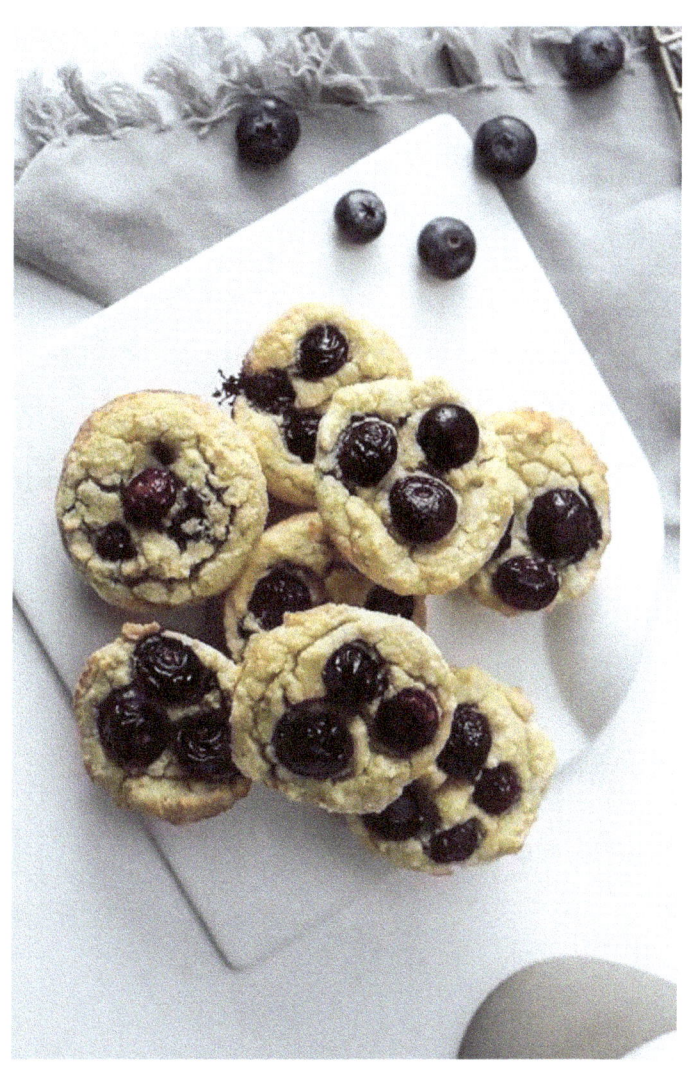

Breakfast Bowl

Preparation time: 10 minutes **Cooking time:** 20 minutes **Servings:** 1

Ingredients:

- 8 mushrooms, sliced
- Salt and black pepper to the taste
- 2 eggs, whisked
- 1 tablespoon coconut oil
- ½ teaspoon smoked paprika
- 1 avocado, pitted, peeled and chopped
- 12 black olives, pitted and sliced
- 4 ounces beef, ground
- 1 yellow onion, chopped

Directions:

Heat up a pan with the coconut oil over medium heat, add onions, mushrooms, salt and pepper, stir and cook for 5 minutes.

2. Add beef and paprika, stir, cook for 10 minutes and transfer to a bowl.

3. Heat up the pan again over medium heat, add eggs, some salt and pepper and scramble them.

4. Return beef mix to pan and stir.

5. Add avocado and olives, stir and cook for 1 minute.

6. Transfer to a bowl and serve.

7. Enjoy!

Nutrition: calories 600, fat 23, fiber 8, carbs 22, protein 43

Low-Carb Cheesecake

Preparation Time: 10 minutes **Cooking Time:** 20 minutes **Servings:** 5

Ingredients:
- 8 oz. of room temp full-fat cream cheese
- 2 Large eggs
- 1 ½ tsp. of granulated stevia/erythritol blend
- ¼ tsp. of pure vanilla extract
- ¼ tsp. of pure almond extract

Kitchen Equipment:
- oven
- muffin tin cups
- cupcake liners

Directions:

1. Warm the oven to 325° Fahrenheit.
2. Prepare five muffin tin cups using cupcake liners.
3. Beat the cream cheese until it's creamy smooth, whisk in the eggs, and the rest of the fixings.
4. Dump the batter into the muffin tins.
5. Set the timer (15–20 minutes) and bake until the cheesecakes are puffy but still wobbly in the center.
6. Cool to room temperature before placing it in the refrigerator to chill for two hours before serving.

Nutrition: Protein: 4g **Total Fats:** 17g - **Calories** 181

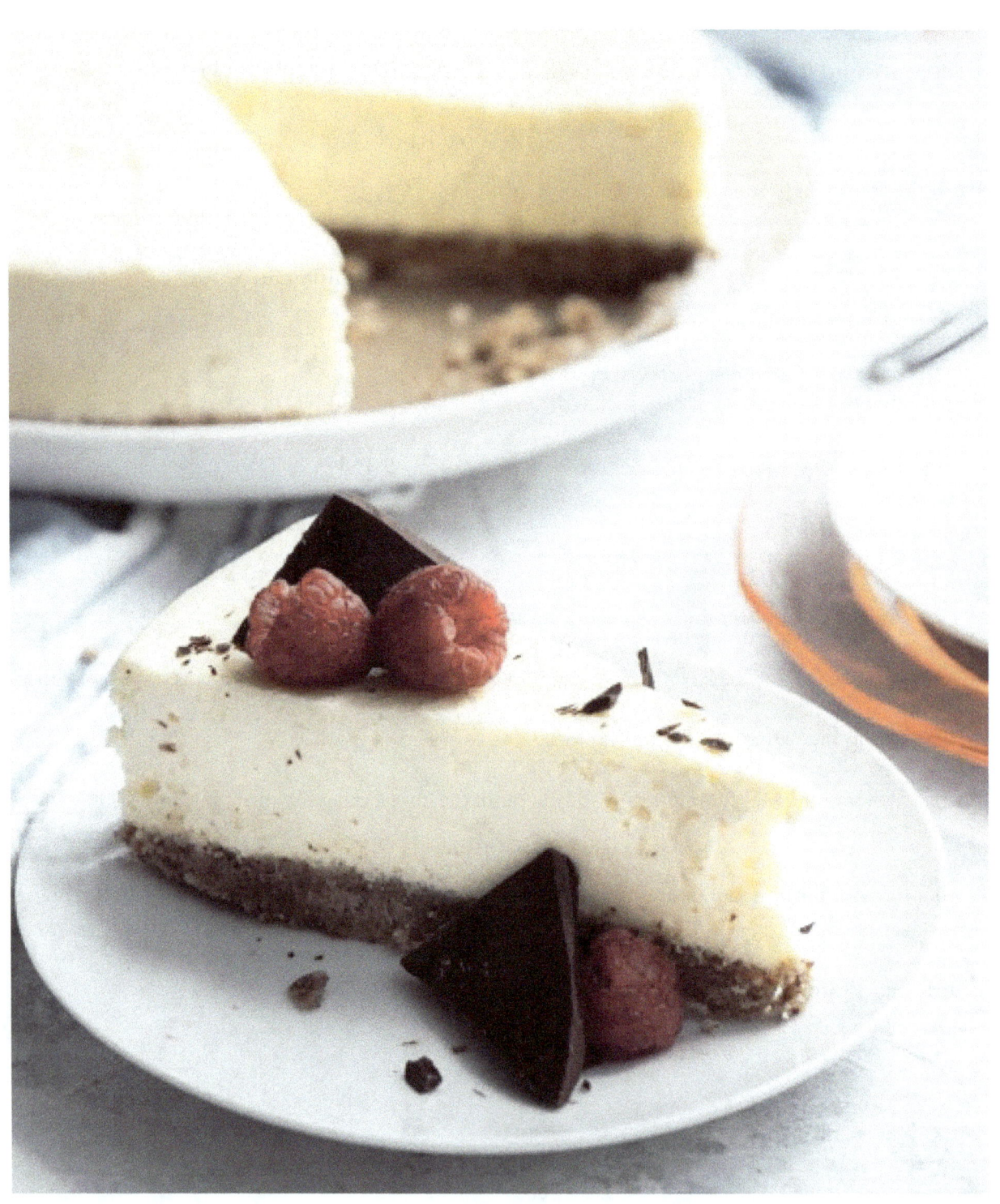

Eggs And Sausages

Preparation time: 10 minutes **Cooking time:** 35 minutes **Servings:** 6

Ingredients:
- 5 tablespoons ghee
- 12 eggs
- Salt and black pepper to the taste 1-ounce spinach, torn
- 12 ham slices
- 2 sausages, chopped
- 1 yellow onion, chopped
- 1 red bell pepper, chopped

Directions:

1. Heat up a pan with 1 tablespoon ghee over medium heat, add sausages and onion, stir and cook for 5 minutes.

2. Add bell pepper, salt and pepper, stir and cook for 3 minutes more and transfer to a bowl.

3. Melt the rest of the ghee and divide into 12 cupcake molds.

4. Add a slice of ham in each cupcake mold, divide spinach in each and then the sausage mix.

5. Crack an egg on top, introduce everything in the oven and bake at 425 degrees F for 20 minutes.

6. Leave your keto cupcakes to cool down a bit before serving.

Enjoy!

Nutrition: calories 440, fat 32, fiber 0, carbs 12, protein 22

Brussels Sprouts Casserole

Gluten Free, Nut Free

Preparation Time: 15 minutes **Cooking Time:** 30 minutes **Servings:** 8

Ingredients:
- 8 bacon slices
- 1-pound of Brussels sprouts (blanched for 10 minutes and cut into quarters)
- 1 cup of shredded Swiss cheese (divided)
- ¾ cup of heavy (whipping) cream

Kitchen Equipment:
- oven
- skillet
- casserole dish
- medium bowl

Directions:

1. Set the oven to 400°F. Situate a skillet over medium-high heat and cook the bacon until it is crispy, about 6 minutes.

2. Set aside 1 tablespoon of bacon fat to grease the casserole dish and roughly chop the cooked bacon. Lightly oil a casserole dish with the reserved bacon fat and set aside.

3. In a medium bowl, toss the Brussels sprouts with the chopped bacon and ½ cup of cheese and transfer the mixture to the casserole dish.

4. Transfer the heavy cream over the Brussels sprouts and top the casserole with the remaining ½ cup of cheese. Bake until the cheese is melted and lightly browned and the vegetables are heated through, about 20 minutes. Serve.

Nutrition: Calories: 299 - **Fat:** 11g - **Protein:** 12g

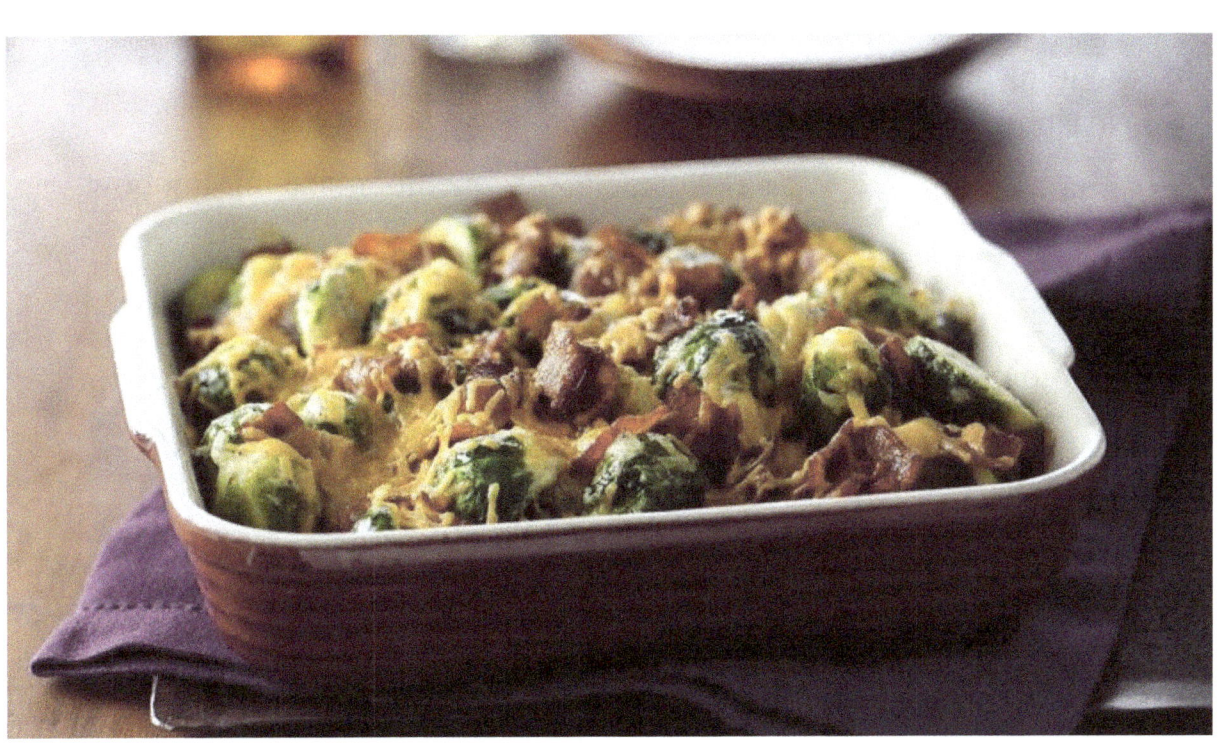

Almond Flour Keto Pancakes

Preparation Time: 10 minutes **Cooking Time:** 12 minutes **Servings:** 10

Ingredients:
- 4 oz. of softened cream cheese, at room temperature
- Zest of 1 medium-sized lemon, fresh (approximately 1 teaspoon)
- 4 large-sized eggs, organic
- ½ cup of almond flour
- 1 tablespoon of butter, for frying and serving

Kitchen Equipment:
- medium-size mixing bowl
- nonstick skillet

Directions:
1. Combine the almond flour with eggs, cream cheese, and lemon zest using a whisk in a medium-sized mixing bowl until combined well, and completely smooth, for a minute or two.
2. The next step is to heat a large, nonstick skillet over medium heat until hot.
3. Once done, add 1 tablespoon of butter until completely melted; swirl to coat the bottom completely.
4. Pour 3 tablespoons of the prepared batter (for each pancake) and cook for a minute or two, until turn golden.
5. Carefully flip, cook the other side for 2 more minutes.
6. Transfer to a clean, large plate and continue cooking with the remaining batter.
7. Top the cooked pancakes with some butter; serve immediately and enjoy.

Nutrition: Calories: 120 - **Total Carbohydrates:** 2g - **Protein:** 3.9g

Ranch Cauliflower Crackers

Preparation Time: 10 minutes **Cooking Time:** 70 minutes **Servings:** 6

Ingredients:
- 12 ounces of cauliflower rice
- Cheesecloth
- 1 large egg
- 1 tbsp. of ranch salad dressing mix (dry)
- 1/8 tsp. of cayenne pepper
- 1 cup of parmesan cheese (shredded)

Kitchen Equipment:
- microwave
- strainer
- oven
- parchment paper
- baking tray

Directions:

1. Add the cauliflower rice in a large bowl.
2. Microwave for four minutes covered.
3. Transfer the cauliflower rice to a strainer lined with cheesecloth.
4. Squeeze out excess moisture.
5. Preheat oven at two hundred degrees Celsius.
6. Use parchment paper for lining a baking tray.
7. Combine egg, cauliflower rice, ranch mix, and pepper in a bowl.
8. Add the cheese.
9. Mix well.

10. Take two tbsps. of the mixture and stir in to the baking tray.

11. Flatten with your hands. The thinner you can make the mixture, the crispier will be the crackers.

12. Bake for ten minutes.

13. Flip the crackers.

14. Bake for ten minutes.

15. Serve warm.

Nutrition: Calories: 29.6 **Protein:** 2.6g **Fat:** 2.6g

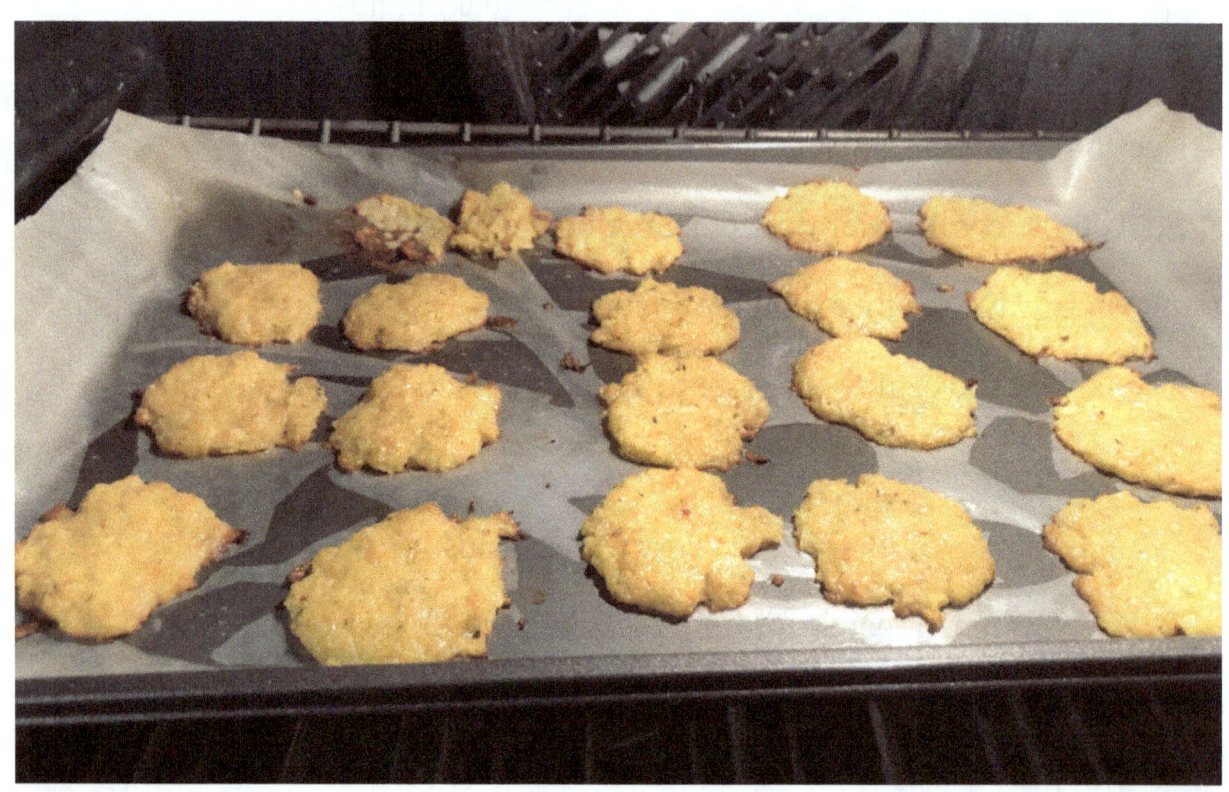

Scrambled Eggs

Preparation time: 10 minutes **Cooking time:** 10 minutes **Servings:** 1

Ingredients:
- 4 bell mushrooms, chopped
- 3 eggs, whisked
- Salt and black pepper to the taste
- 2 ham slices, chopped
- ¼ cup red bell pepper, chopped
- ½ cup spinach, chopped
- 1 tablespoon coconut oil

Directions:
1. Heat up a pan with half of the oil over medium heat, add mushrooms, spinach, ham and bell pepper, stir and cook for 4 minutes.
2. Heat up another pan with the rest of the oil over medium heat, add eggs and scramble them.
3. Add veggies and ham, salt and pepper, stir, cook for 1 minute and serve.
4. Enjoy!

Nutrition: calories 350, fat 23, fiber 1, carbs 5, protein 22

Frittata

Preparation time: 10 minutes **Cooking time:** 1 hour **Servings:**

Ingredients:

- A pinch of nutmeg
- 4 tablespoons olive oil
- 9 ounces spinach
- 12 eggs
- 1-ounce pepperoni
- 1 teaspoon garlic, minced
- Salt and black pepper to the taste
- 5 ounces mozzarella, shredded
- ½ cup parmesan, grated
- ½ cup ricotta cheese

Directions:

1 Squeeze liquid from spinach and put in a bowl.

2 In another bowl, mix eggs with salt, pepper, nutmeg and garlic and whisk well.

3 Add spinach, parmesan and ricotta and whisk well again.

4 Pour this into a pan, sprinkle mozzarella and pepperoni on top, introduce in the oven and bake at 375 degrees F for 45 minutes.

5 Leave frittata to cool down for a few minutes before serving it.

5. Enjoy!

Nutrition: calories 298, fat 2, fiber 1, carbs 6, protein 18

Smoked Salmon Breakfast

Preparation time: 10 minutes **Cooking time:** 10 minutes **Servings:** 3

Ingredients:

- Salt and black pepper to the taste
- 1 tablespoon lemon juice
- ¼ cup green onions, chopped
- 1 teaspoon garlic powder
- *For the sauce:*
- 1 cup coconut milk
- ½ cup cashews, soaked, drained
- 4 eggs, whisked
- ½ teaspoon avocado oil
- 4 ounces smoked salmon, chopped

Directions:

1. In your blender, mix cashews with coconut milk, garlic powder and lemon juice and blend well.

2. Add salt, pepper and green onions, blend again well, transfer to a bowl and keep in the fridge for now.

3. Heat up a pan with the oil over medium-low heat, add eggs, whisk a bit and cook until they are almost done

4. Introduce in your preheated broiler and cook until eggs set.

5. Divide eggs on plates, top with smoked salmon and serve with the green onion sauce on top.

Enjoy!

Nutrition: calories 200, fat 10, fiber 2, carbs 11, protein 15

Breakfast Eggs

Preparation time: 10 minutes **Cooking time:** 4 minutes **Servings:** 12

Ingredients:
- 1 tablespoons peppercorns
- 8 cups water
- 1 cup tamari sauce
- 2 tablespoons cinnamon 6-star anise
- 1 teaspoon black pepper
- 4 tea bags
- 4 tablespoons salt
- 12 eggs

Directions:
1. Put water in a pot, add eggs, bring them to a boil over medium heat and cook until they are hard boiled.
2. Cool them down and crack them without peeling.
3. In a large pot, mix water with tea bags, salt, pepper, peppercorns, cinnamon, star anise and tamari sauce.
4. Add cracked eggs, cover pot, bring to a simmer over low heat and cook for 30 minutes.
5. Discard tea bags and cook eggs for 3 hours and 30 minutes.
6. Leave eggs to cool down, peel and serve them for breakfast.

Enjoy!

Nutrition: calories 90, fat 6, fiber 0, carbs 0, protein 7

Eggs Baked In Avocados

Preparation time: 10 minutes **Cooking time:** 20 minutes **Servings:** 4

Ingredients:

- Salt and black pepper to the taste
- 1 tablespoon chives, chopped
- 2 avocados, cut in halves and pitted
- 4 eggs

Directions:

1. Scoop some flesh from the avocado halves and arrange them in a baking dish.
2. Crack an egg in each avocado, season with salt and pepper, introduce them in the oven at 425 degrees F and bake for 20 minutes.
3. Sprinkle chives at the end and serve for breakfast!

Enjoy!

Nutrition: calories 400, fat 34, fiber 13, carbs 13, protein 15

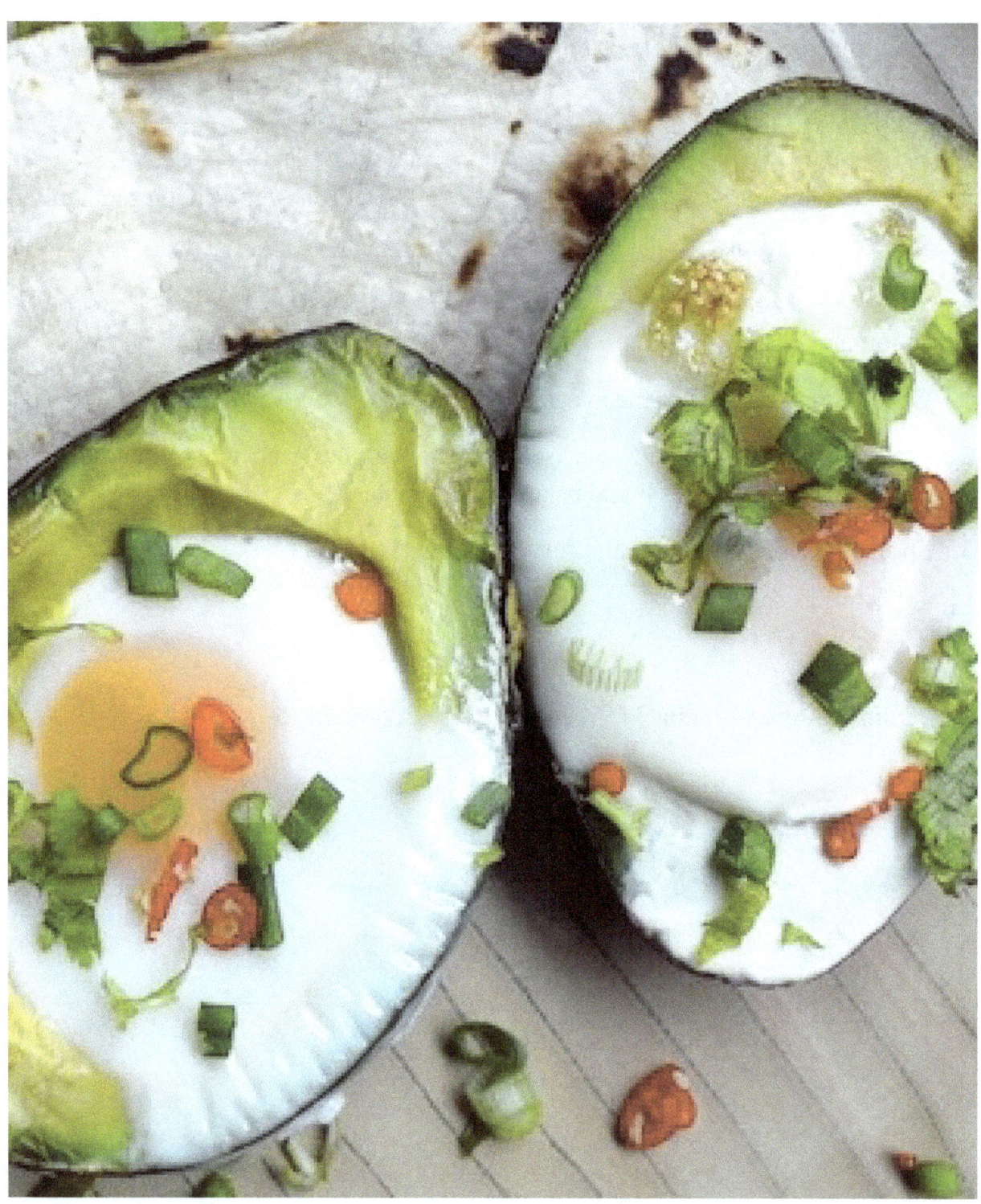

Bacon Breakfast And Shrimp

Preparation time: 10 minutes **Cooking time:** 15 minutes **Servings:** 4

Ingredients:

- Salt and black pepper to the taste
- ½ cup coconut cream
- 4 bacon slices, chopped
- 4 ounces smoked salmon, chopped
- 4 ounces shrimp, deveined
- 1 cup mushrooms, sliced

Directions:

1. Heat up a pan over medium heat, add bacon, stir and cook for 5 minutes.
2. Add mushrooms, stir and cook for 5 minutes more.
3. Add salmon, stir and cook for 3 minutes.
4. Add shrimp and cook for 2 minutes.
5. Add salt, pepper and coconut cream, stir, cook for 1 minute, take off heat and divide between plates.

Enjoy!

Nutrition: calories 340, fat 23, fiber 1, carbs 4, protein 17

Breakfast Pie

Preparation time: 10 minutes **Cooking time:** 45 minutes **Servings:** 8

Ingredients:
- Mango salsa for serving
- 1 teaspoon baking soda
- A handful cilantro, chopped
- 8 eggs
- 1 teaspoon coconut oil
- ¾ pound beef, ground
- Salt and black pepper to the taste
- 3 tablespoons taco seasoning
- ½ onion, chopped
- 1 pie crust
- ½ red bell pepper, chopped

Directions:

1. Heat up a pan with the oil over medium heat, add beef, cook until it browns and mixes with salt, pepper and taco seasoning.

2. Stir again, transfer to a bowl and leave aside for now.

3. Heat up the pan again over medium heat with cooking juices from the meat, add onion and bell pepper, stir and cook for 4 minutes.

4. Add eggs, baking soda and some salt and stir well.

5. Add cilantro, stir again and take off heat.

6. Spread beef mix in pie crust, add veggies mix and spread over meat, introduce in the oven at 350 degrees F and bake for 45 minutes.

7. Leave the pie to cool down a bit, slice, divide between plates and serve with mango salsa on top.

Enjoy!

Nutrition: calories 198, fat 11, fiber 1, carbs 12, protein 12

Mexican Breakfast

Preparation time: 10 minutes **Cooking time:** 30 minutes **Servings:** 8

Ingredients:
- ½ cup red onion, chopped
- 1 avocado, pitted, peeled and chopped
- 3 tablespoons ghee
- Salt and black pepper to the taste
- 8 eggs
- 1 tomato, chopped
- ½ cup enchilada sauce
- 1 pound pork, ground
- 1 pound chorizo, chopped

Directions:
1. In a bowl, mix pork with chorizo, stir and spread on a lined baking form.
2. Spread enchilada sauce on top, introduce in the oven at 350 degrees F and bake for 20 minutes.
3. Heat up a pan with the ghee over medium heat, add eggs and scramble them well.
4. Take pork mix out of the oven and spread scrambled eggs over them.
5. Sprinkle salt, pepper, tomato, onion and avocado, divide between plates and serve.

Enjoy!

Nutrition: calories 400, fat 32, fiber 4, carbs 7, protein 25

Breakfast Stir Fry

Preparation time: 10 minutes **Cooking time:** 30 minutes **Servings:** 2

Ingredients:
- 1 teaspoon chili powder
- 1 tablespoon coconut oil
- Salt and black pepper to the taste
- 1 tablespoon tamari sauce
- 2 bell peppers, chopped
- ½ pounds beef meat, minced
- 2 teaspoons red chili flake
- 6 bunches bok choy, trimmed and chopped
- 1 teaspoon ginger, grated Salt to the taste
- 1 tablespoon coconut oil
- 1 tablespoon coconut oil
- 2 eggs

Directions:
1. Heat up a pan with 1 tablespoon coconut oil over medium high heat, add beef and bell peppers, stir and cook for 10 minutes.
2. Add salt, pepper, tamari sauce, chili flakes and chili powder, stir, cook for 4 minutes more and take off heat.
3. Heat up another pan with 1 tablespoon oil over medium heat, add bok choy, stir and cook for 3 minutes.
4. Add salt and ginger, stir, cook for 2 minutes more and take off heat.
5. Heat up the third pan with 1 tablespoon oil over medium heat, crack eggs and fry them.
6. Divide beef and bell peppers mix into 2 bowls.
7. Divide bok choy and top with eggs.
8. Enjoy!

Nutrition: calories 248, fat 14, fiber 4, carbs 10, protein 14

Breakfast Casserole

Preparation time: 10 minutes **Cooking time:** 40 minutes **Servings:** 4

- **Ingredients:**
- 3 cups spinach, torn
- Salt and black pepper to the taste
- 3 tablespoons avocado oil
- 1 pound pork sausage, chopped
- 1 yellow onion, chopped
- 10 eggs

Directions:

1. Heat up a pan with 1 tablespoon oil over medium heat, add sausage, stir and brown it for 4 minutes.
2. Add onion, stir and cook for 3 minutes more.
3. Add spinach, stir and cook for 1 minute.
4. Grease a baking dish with the rest of the oil and spread sausage mix.
5. Whisk eggs and add them to sausage mix.
6. Stir gently, introduce in the oven at 350 degrees F and bake for 30 minutes.
7. Leave casserole to cool down for a few minutes before serving it for breakfast.

Enjoy!

Nutrition: calories 345, fat 12, fiber 1, carbs 8, protein 22

Breakfast Skillet

Preparation time: 10 minutes **Cooking time:** 30 minutes **Servings:** 4

Ingredients:
- teaspoon basil, dried
- 2 tablespoons Dijon mustard
- 2 zucchinis, chopped
- teaspoon basil, dried
- 2 tablespoons Dijon mustard
- 2 zucchinis, chopped
- 8 ounces mushrooms, chopped
- Salt and black pepper to the taste
- 1 pound pork, minced

Directions:
1. Heat up a pan with the oil over medium high heat, add mushrooms, stir and cook for 4 minutes.
2. Add zucchinis, salt and pepper, stir and cook for 4 minutes more.
3. Add pork, garlic powder, basil, more salt and pepper, stir and cook until meat is done.
4. Add mustard, stir, cook for 3 minutes more, divide into bowls and serve.

Enjoy!

Nutrition: calories 240, fat 15, fiber 2, carbs 9, protein 17

Breakfast Dish

Preparation time: 10 minutes **Cooking time:** 40 minutes **Servings:** 6

Ingredients:
- 1 tablespoon dill, chopped
- Salt and black pepper to the taste
- ¼ teaspoon garlic powder
- 1 tablespoon coconut oil, melted
- 8 eggs, whisked
- ¼ cup coconut milk
- 1 pound sausage, chopped

1 leek, chopped

Directions:
1. Heat up a pan over medium heat, add sausage pieces and brown them for a few minutes.
2. Add asparagus and leek, stir and cook for a few minutes.
3. Meanwhile, in a bowl, mix eggs with salt, pepper, dill, garlic powder and coconut milk and whisk well.
4. Pour this into a baking dish which you've greased with the coconut oil.
5. Add sausage and veggies on top and whisk everything.
6. Introduce in the oven at 325 degrees F and bake for 40 minutes.
7. Serve warm.

Enjoy!

Nutrition: calories 340, fat 12, fiber 3, carbs 8, protein 23

Breakfast Patties

Preparation time: 10 minutes **Cooking time:** 10 minutes **Servings:** 4

Ingredients:
- ¼ teaspoon ginger, dried
- 3 tablespoon cold water
- 1 tablespoon coconut oil
- ½ teaspoon sage, dried
- Salt and black pepper to the taste
- ¼ teaspoon thyme, dried
- 1 pound pork meat, minced

Directions:
1. Put meat in a bowl.
2. In another bowl, mix water with salt, pepper, sage, thyme and ginger and whisk well.
3. Add this to meat and stir very well.
4. Shape your patties and place them on a working surface.
5. Heat up a pan with the coconut oil over medium high heat, add patties, fry them for 5 minutes, flip and cook them for 3 minutes more.
6. Serve them warm.

Enjoy!

Nutrition: calories 320, fat 13, fiber 2, carbs 10, protein 12

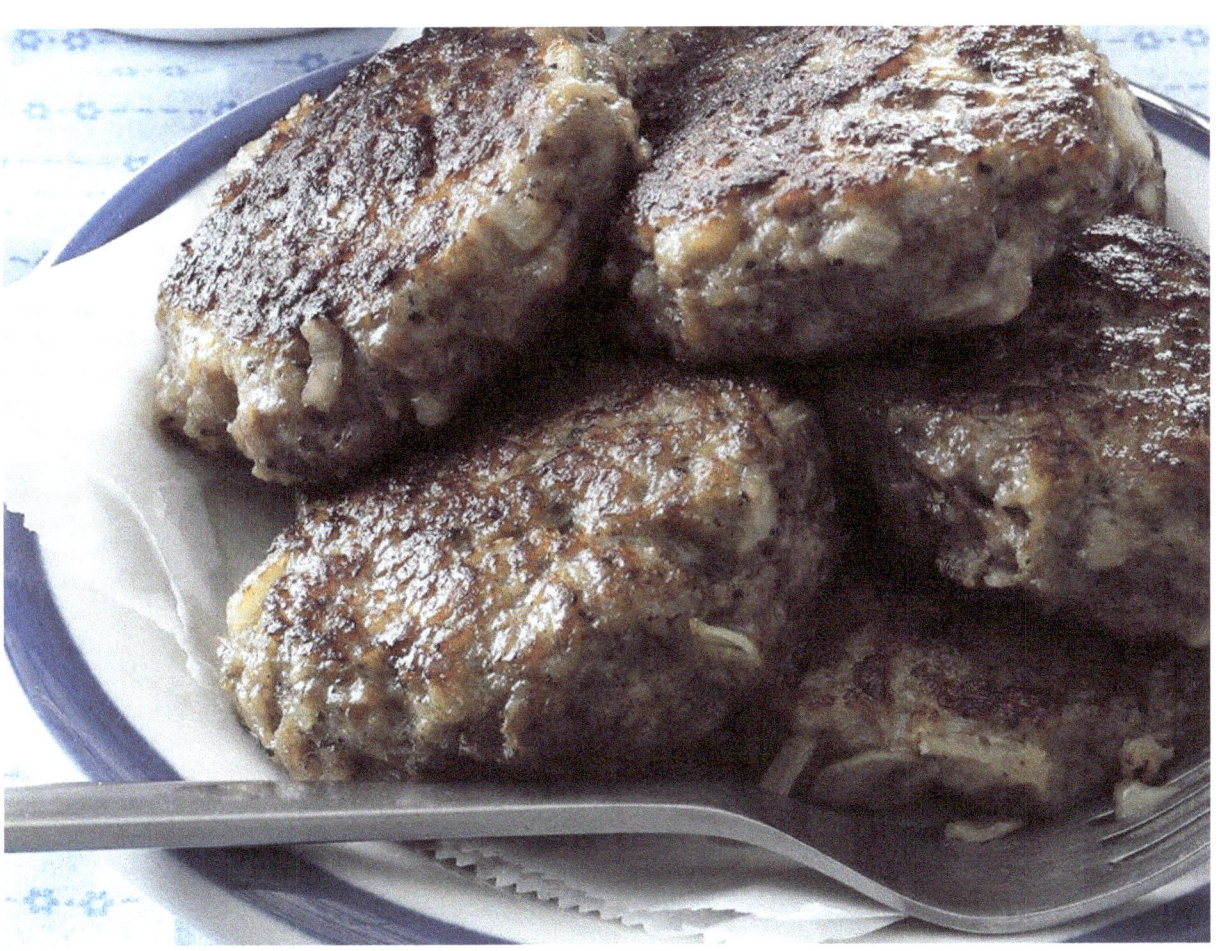

Sausage Quiche

Preparation time: 10 minutes **Cooking time:** 40 minutes **Servings:** 6

Ingredients:
- 2 teaspoons whipping cream
- 2 tablespoons parsley, chopped
- Salt and black pepper to the taste
- 12 ounces pork sausage, chopped
- 10 mixed cherry tomatoes, halved
- 5 eggplant slice
- 2 tablespoons parmesan, grated

Directions:
1. Spread sausage pieces on the bottom of a baking dish.
2. Layer eggplant slices on top.
3. Add cherry tomatoes.
4. In a bowl, mix eggs with salt, pepper, cream and parmesan and whisk well.
5. Pour this into the baking dish, introduce in the oven at 375 degrees F and bake for 40 minutes.
6. Serve right away.

Enjoy!

Nutrition: calories 340, fat 28, fiber 3, carbs 3, protein 17

Cauliflower Breakfast and Chorizo

Preparation time: 10 minutes **Cooking time:** 45 minutes **Servings:** 4

Ingredients:

- 4 eggs, whisked
- 2 tablespoons green onions, chopped
- Salt and black pepper to the taste
- 1 cauliflower head, florets separated
- 1 yellow onion, chopped ½ teaspoon garlic powder
- 12 ounces canned green chilies, chopped
- 1 pound chorizo, chopped

Directions:

1. Heat up a pan over medium heat, add chorizo and onion, stir and brown for a few minutes.
2. Add green chilies, stir, cook for a few minutes and take off heat.
3. In your food processor mix cauliflower with some salt and pepper and blend.
4. Transfer this to a bowl, add eggs, salt, pepper and garlic powder and whisk everything.
5. Add chorizo mix as well, whisk again and transfer everything to a greased baking dish.
6. Bake in the oven at 375 degrees F and bake for 40 minutes.
7. Leave casserole to cool down for a few minutes, sprinkle green onions on top, slice and serve.

Enjoy!

Nutrition: calories 350, fat 12, fiber 4, carbs 6, protein 20

Breakfast Porridge

Preparation time: 5 minutes **Cooking time:** 10 minutes **Servings:** 1

Ingredients:
- 1 teaspoon cinnamon powder
- A pinch of nutmeg
- A pinch of cardamom, ground
- A pinch of cloves, ground
- ½ cup almonds, ground
- 1 teaspoon stevia
- ¾ cup coconut cream

Directions:
1. Heat up a pan over medium heat, add coconut cream and heat up for a few minutes.
2. Add stevia and almonds and stir well for 5 minutes.
3. Add cloves, cardamom, nutmeg and cinnamon and stir well.
4. Transfer to a bowl and serve hot.

Enjoy!

Nutrition: calories 200, fat 12, fiber 4, carbs 8, protein 16

Italian Spaghetti Casserole

Preparation time: 10 minutes **Cooking time:** 10 minutes **Servings:** 4

Ingredients:
- ½ cup kalamata olives, chopped
- 4 eggs
- A handful parsley, chopped
- ½ teaspoon Italian seasoning
- 3 ounces Italian salami, chopped
- 2 garlic cloves, minced
- 1 cup yellow onion, chopped
- Salt and black pepper to the taste
- ½ cup tomatoes, chopped
- 4 tablespoons ghee
- 1 squash, halved

Directions:
1. Place squash halves on a lined baking sheet, season with salt and pepper, spread 1 tablespoon ghee over them, introduce in the oven at 400 degrees F and bake for 45 minutes.
2. Meanwhile, heat up a pan with the rest of the ghee over medium heat, add garlic, onions, salt and pepper, stir and cook for a couple of minutes.
3. Add salami and tomatoes, stir and cook for 10 minutes.
4. Add olives, stir and cook for a few minutes more.
5. Take squash halves out of the oven, scrape flesh with a fork and add over salami mix into the pan.
6. Stir, make 4 holes in the mix, crack an egg in each, season with salt and pepper, introduce pan in the oven at 400 degrees F and bake until eggs are done.7. Sprinkle parsley on top and serve.

Enjoy!

Nutrition: calories 333, fat 23, fiber 4, carbs 12, protein 15

Granola

Preparation time: 10 minutes **Cooking time:** 0 minutes **Servings:** 2

Ingredients:
- A splash of lemon juice
- 2 tablespoons pecans, chopped
- 2 tablespoons chocolate, chopped
- 7 strawberries, chopped

Directions:
1. In a bowl, mix chocolate with strawberries, pecans and lemon juice.
2. Stir and serve cold.

Enjoy!

Nutrition: calories 200, fat 5, fiber 4, carbs 7, protein 8

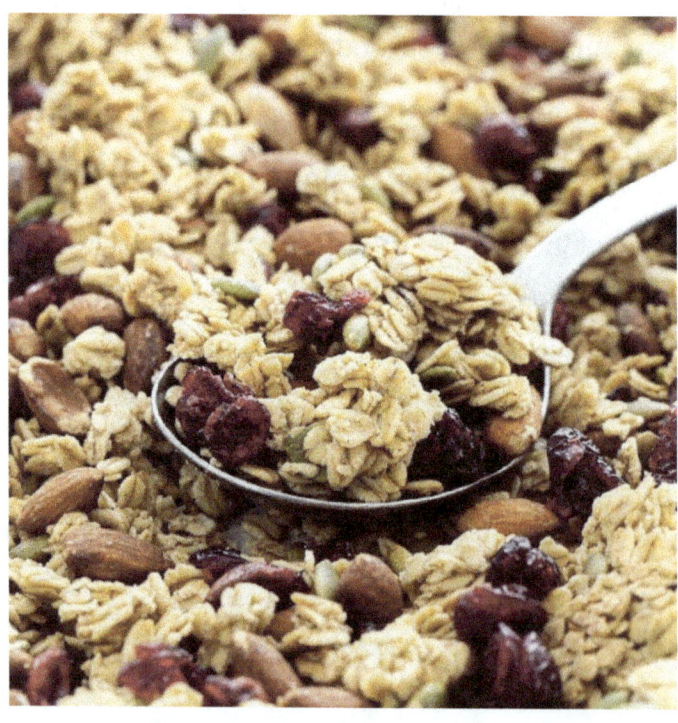

Breakfast Bowl

Preparation time: 5 minutes **Cooking time:** 0 minutes **Servings:** 1

Ingredients:

- 1 teaspoon pepitas, raw
- 2 teaspoons raspberries
- 1 teaspoon sunflower seeds, raw
- 1 teaspoon raw honey
- 1 teaspoon almonds, chopped
- 1 teaspoon pine nuts, raw
- 1 teaspoon pistachios, chopped
- 1 cup coconut milk
- 1 teaspoon walnuts, chopped
- 1 teaspoon pecans, chopped

Directions:

In a bowl, mix milk with honey and stir.

2. Add pecans, walnuts, almonds, pistachios, sunflower seeds, pine nuts and pepitas.

3. Stir, top with raspberries and serve.

Enjoy!

Nutrition: calories 100, fat 2, fiber 4, carbs 5, protein 6

Almond Cereal

Preparation time: 5 minutes **Cooking time:** 0 minutes. **Servings:** 1

Ingredients:
- A handful blueberries
- 1 small banana, chopped
- 1 tablespoon chia seeds
- 1/3 cup water
- 2 tablespoon pepitas, roasted
- 1/3 cup coconut milk
- 2 tablespoons almonds, chopped

Directions:
1. In a bowl, mix chia seeds with coconut milk and leave aside for 5 minutes.
2. In your food processor, mix half of the pepitas with almonds and pulse them well.
3. Add this to chia seeds mix.
4. Also add the water and stir.
5. Top with the rest of the pepitas, banana pieces and blueberries and serve.

Enjoy!

Nutrition: calories 200, fat 3, fiber 2, carbs 5, protein 4

Breakfast Bread

Preparation time: 10 minutes **Cooking time:** 3 minutes **Servings:** 4

Ingredients:

- 2 and ½ tablespoons coconut oil
- 1 egg, whisked
- A pinch of salt
- 1/3 cup almond flour
- ½ teaspoon baking powder

Directions:

1. Grease a mug with some of the oil.
2. In a bowl, mix the egg with flour, salt, oil and baking powder and stir.
3. Pour this into the mug and cook in your microwave for 3 minutes at a High temperature.
4. Leave the bread to cool down a bit, take out of the mug, slice and serve with a glass of almond milk for breakfast.

Enjoy!

Nutrition: calories 132, fat 12, fiber 1, carbs 3, protein 4

Breakfast Muffins

Preparation time: 10 minutes **Cooking time:** 30 minutes **Servings:** 4

Ingredients:

- 8 prosciutto slices
- ¼ cup chives, chopped
- Salt and black pepper to the taste
- 6 eggs
- ¼ cup kale, chopped
- 1 tablespoon coconut oil
- ½ cup almond milk

Directions:

1. In a bowl, mix eggs with salt, pepper, milk, chives and kale and stir well.
2. Grease a muffin tray with melted coconut oil, line with prosciutto slices, pour eggs mix, introduce in the oven and bake at 350 degrees F for 30 minutes.
3. Transfer muffins to a platter and serve for breakfast.

Enjoy!

Nutrition: calories 140, fat 3, fiber 1, carbs 3, protein 10

Chicken Breakfast Muffins

Preparation time: 10 minutes **Cooking time:** 1 hour **Servings:** 3

Ingredients:
- 6 eggs
- 2 tablespoons green onions, chopped
- 3 tablespoons hot sauce mixed with 3 tablespoons melted coconut oil
- ½ teaspoon garlic powder
- Salt and black pepper to the taste
- ¾ pound chicken breast, boneless

Directions:
1. Season chicken breast with salt, pepper and garlic powder, place on a lined baking sheet and bake in the oven at 425 degrees F for 25 minutes.
2. Transfer chicken breast to a bowl, shred with a fork and mix with half of the hot sauce and melted coconut oil.
3. Toss to coat and leave aside for now.
4. In a bowl, mix eggs with salt, pepper, green onions and the rest of the hot sauce mixed with oil and whisk very well.
5. Divide this mix into a muffin tray, top each with shredded chicken, introduce in the oven at 350 degrees F and bake for 30 minutes.
6. Serve your muffins hot.

Enjoy!

Nutrition: calories 140, fat 8, fiber 1, carbs 2, protein 13

Breakfast Sandwich

Preparation time: 10 minutes **Cooking time:** 10 minutes **Servings:** 1

Ingredients:
- 2 eggs
- 2 tablespoons ghee
- Salt and black pepper to the taste
- 1 tablespoon guacamole
- ¼ cup water
- ¼ pound pork sausage meat, minced

Directions:
1. In a bowl, mix minced sausage meat with salt and pepper to the taste and stir well.
2. Shape a patty from this mix and place on a working surface.
3. Heat up a pan with 1 tablespoon ghee over medium heat, add sausage patty, fry for 3 minutes on each side and transfer to a plate.
4. Crack an egg in 2 bowls and whisk them a bit with some salt and pepper.
5. Heat up a pan with the rest of the ghee over medium high heat, place 2 biscuit cutters which you've greased with some ghee before in the pan and pour an egg in each.
6. Add the water to the pan, reduce heat, cover pan and cook eggs for 3 minutes.
7. Transfer these egg "buns" to paper towels and drain grease.
8. Place sausage patty on one egg "bun" spread guacamole over it and top with the other egg "bun".

Enjoy!

Nutrition: calories 200, fat 4, fiber 6, carbs 5, protein 10

Avocado Muffins

Preparation time: 10 minutes **Cooking time:** 20 minutes **Servings:** 12

Ingredients:
- ½ cup coconut flour
- 2 cups avocado, pitted, peeled and chopped
- Salt and black pepper to the taste
- ½ teaspoon baking soda
- 1 cup coconut milk
- 1 yellow onion, chopped
- 4 eggs
- 6 bacon slices, chopped

Directions:
1. Heat up a pan over medium heat, add onion and bacon, stir and brown for a few minutes.
2. In a bowl, mash avocado pieces with a fork and whisk well with the eggs.
3. Add milk, salt, pepper, baking soda and coconut flour and stir everything.
4. Add bacon mix and stir again.
5. Grease a muffin tray with the coconut oil, divide eggs and avocado mix into the tray, introduce in the oven at 350 degrees F and bake for 20 minutes.
6. Divide muffins between plates and serve them for breakfast.

Enjoy!

Nutrition: calories 200, fat 7, fiber 4, carbs 7, protein 5

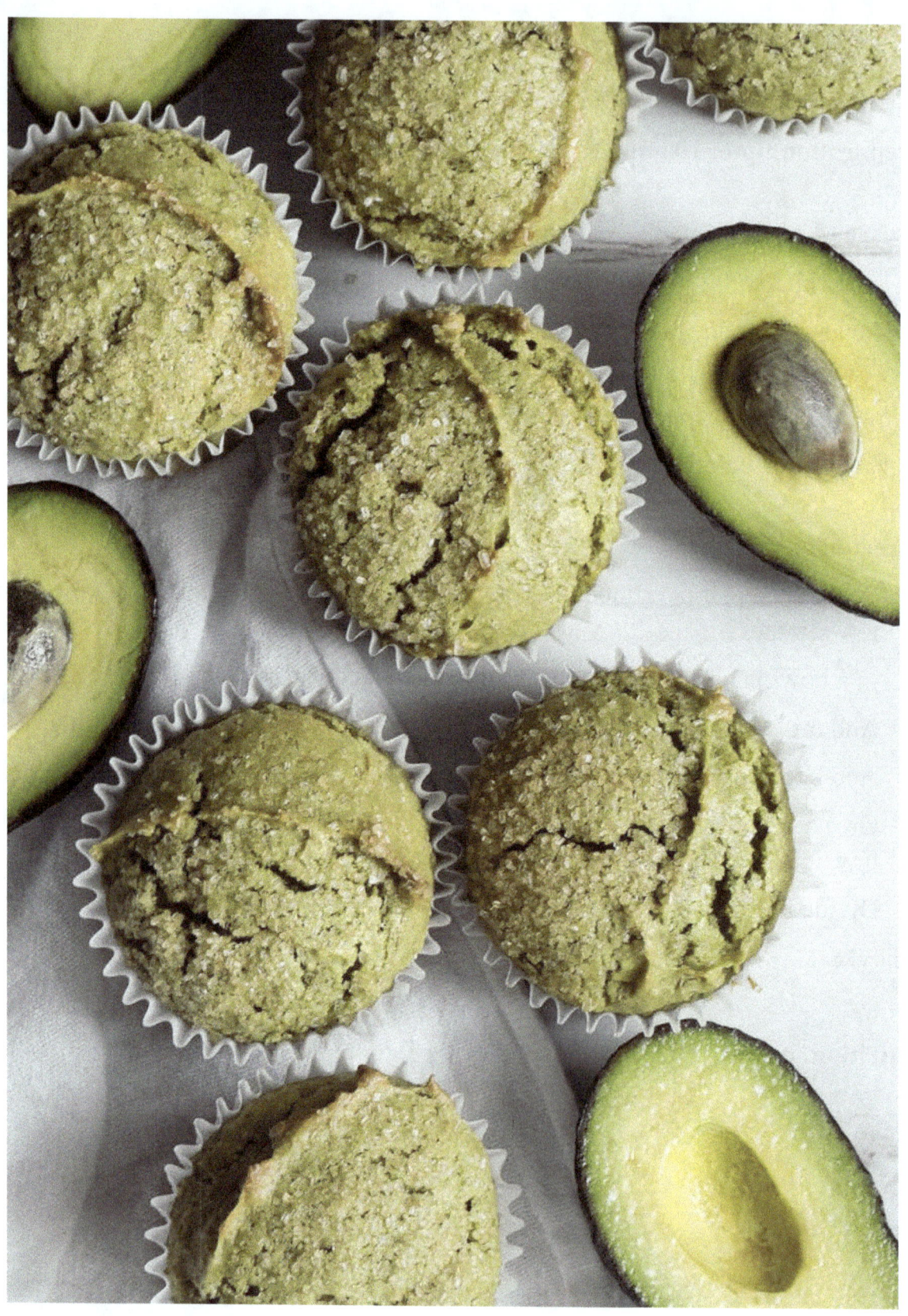

Herbed Biscuits

Preparation time: 10 minutes **Cooking time:** 15 minutes **Servings:** 6

Ingredients:
- ½ teaspoon apple cider vinegar
- ¼ teaspoon baking soda
- 1 tablespoons parsley, chopped
- 2 tablespoons coconut milk
- 2 eggs
- Salt and black pepper to the taste
- ¼ cup yellow onion, minced
- 2 garlic cloves, minced
- 6 tablespoons coconut flour
- 6 tablespoons coconut oil

Directions:
1. In a bowl, mix coconut flour with eggs, oil, garlic, onion, coconut milk, parsley, salt and pepper and stir well.
2. In a bowl, mix vinegar with baking soda, stir well and add to the batter.
3. Drop spoonful of this batter on lined baking sheets and shape circles.
4. Introduce in the oven at 350 degrees F and bake for 17 minutes.
5. Serve these biscuits for breakfast.

Enjoy!

Nutrition: calories 140, fat 6, fiber 2, carbs 10, protein 12

Bacon And Lemon Breakfast Muffins

Preparation time: 10 minutes **Cooking time:** 20 minutes **Servings:** 12

Ingredients:
- 4 eggs
- 2 teaspoons lemon thyme
- 1 teaspoon baking soda
- 3 cups almond flour
- Salt and black pepper to the taste
- ½ cup ghee, melted
- 1 cup bacon, finely chopped

Directions:
1. In a bowl, mix flour with baking soda and eggs and stir well.
2. Add ghee, lemon thyme, bacon, salt and pepper and whisk well.
3. Divide this into a lined muffin pan, introduce in the oven at 350 degrees F and bake for 20 minutes.
4. Leave muffins to cool down a bit, divide between plates and serve them.

Enjoy!

Nutrition: calories 213, fat 7, fiber 2, carbs 9, protein 8

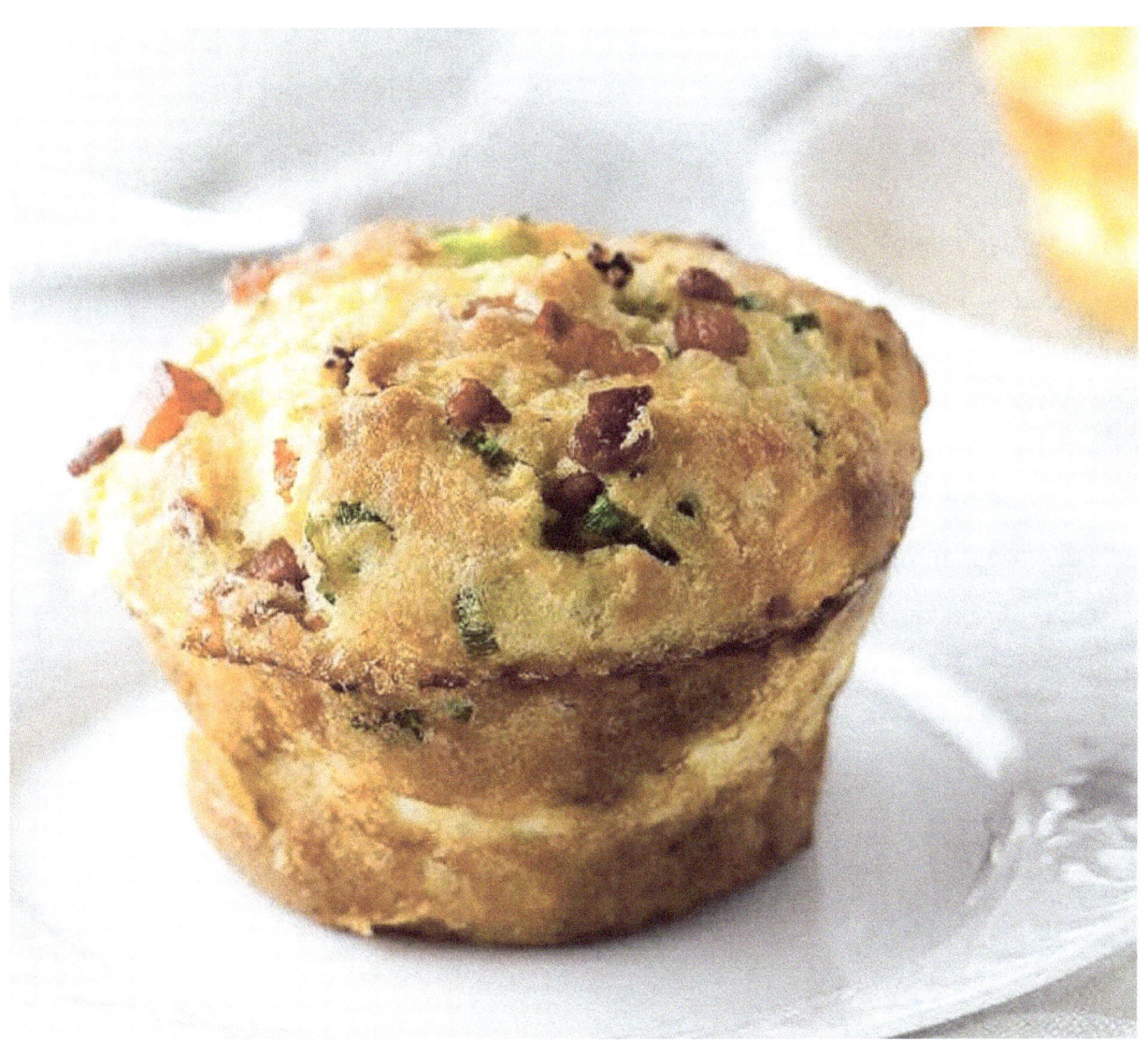

Turkey Breakfast

Preparation time: 10 minutes **Cooking time:** 20 minutes **Servings:** 1

Ingredients:
- 2 tablespoons coconut oil
- 2 eggs, whisked
- 2 tablespoons coconut oil
- 2 eggs, whisked
- Salt and black pepper
- 2 avocado slices

Directions:
1. Heat up a pan over medium heat, add bacon slices and brown them for a few minutes.
2. Meanwhile, heat up another pan with the oil over medium heat, add eggs, salt and pepper and scramble them.
3. Divide turkey breast slices on 2 plates.
4. Divide scrambled eggs on each.
5. Divide bacon slices and avocado slices as well and serve.

Enjoy!

Nutrition: calories 135, fat 7, fiber 2, carbs 4, protein 10

Breakfast Hash

Preparation time: 10 minutes **Cooking time:** 16 minutes **Servings:** 2

Ingredients:
- 2 cups corned beef, chopped
- 1 pound radishes, cut in quarters
- Salt and black pepper to the taste
- 1 yellow onion, chopped
- ½ cup beef stock
- 1 tablespoon coconut oil
- 2 garlic cloves, minced

Directions:
1. Heat up a pan with the oil over medium high heat, add onion, stir and cook for 4 minutes.
2. Add radishes, stir and cook for 5 minutes.
3. Add garlic, stir and cook for 1 minute more.
4. Add stock, beef, salt and pepper, stir, cook for 5 minutes, take off heat and serve.

Enjoy!

Nutrition: calories 240, fat 7, fiber 3, carbs 12, protein 8

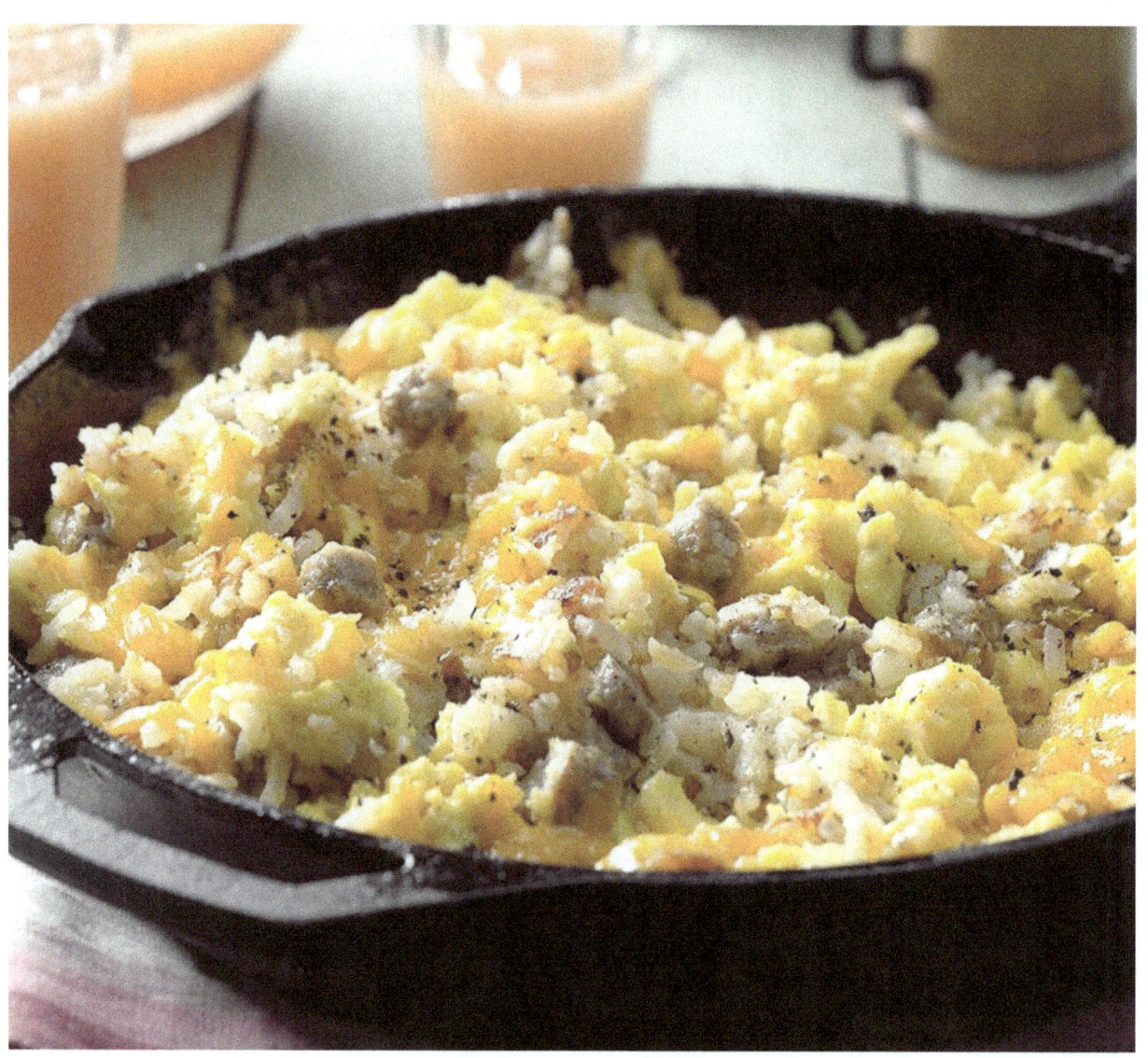

Cocoa Cereal Nibs Breakfast

Preparation time: 10 minutes **Cooking time:** 45 minutes **Servings:** 4

Ingredients:

- 2 tablespoons coconut oil
- 1 tablespoon swerve
- 2 tablespoons cocoa nibs
- 1 tablespoon vanilla extract
- 1 tablespoon psyllium powder
- ½ cup chia seeds
- 1 cup water
- 4 tablespoons hemp hearts

Directions:

1. In a bowl, mix chia seeds with water, stir and leave aside for 5 minutes.
2. Add hemp hearts, vanilla extract, psyllium powder, oil and swerve and stir well with your mixer.
3. Add cocoa nibs, and stir until you obtain a dough.
4. Divide dough into 2 pieces, shape into cylinder form, place on a lined baking sheet, flatten well, cover with a parchment paper, introduce in the oven at 285 degrees F and bake for 20 minutes.
5. Remove the parchment paper and bake for 25 minutes more.
6. Take cylinders out of the oven, leave aside to cool down and cut into small pieces.
7. Serve in the morning with some almond milk.

Enjoy!

Nutrition: calories 245, fat 12, fiber 12, carbs 2, protein 9

Chia Pudding Breakfast

Preparation time: 10 minutes **Cooking time:** 30 minutes **Servings:** 2

Ingredients:
- 1 tablespoon swerve
- 1 tablespoon vanilla extract
- 1/3 cup coconut cream
- 2 tablespoons cocoa nibs
- 1/3 cup chia seeds
- 2 tablespoons coffee
- 2 cups water

Directions:
1. Heat up a small pot with the water over medium heat, bring to a boil, add coffee, simmer for 15 minutes, take off heat and strain into a bowl.
2. Add vanilla extract, coconut cream, swerve, cocoa nibs and chia seeds, stir well, keep in the fridge for 30 minutes, divide into 2 breakfast bowls and serve.

Enjoy!

Nutrition: calories 100, fat 0.4, fiber 4, carbs 3, protein 3

Easy Cereal Breakfast

Preparation time: 10 minutes **Cooking time:** 3 minutes **Servings:** 2

Ingredients:
- A pinch of salt
- 1/3 cup flax seed
- 1/3 cup walnuts, chopped
- 1 tablespoon stevia
- 2 cups almond milk
- ½ cup coconut, shredded
- 4 teaspoons ghee
- 1/3 cup macadamia nuts, chopped

Directions:
1. Heat up a pot with the ghee over medium heat, add milk, coconut, salt, macadamia nuts, walnuts, flax seed and stevia and stir well.
2. Cook for 3 minutes, stir again, take off heat and leave aside for 10 minutes.
3. Divide into 2 bowls and serve.

Enjoy!

Nutrition: calories 140, fat 3, fiber 2, carbs 1.5, protein 7

Sweet Pancakes

Preparation time: 3 minutes **Cooking time:** 12 minutes **Servings:** 4

Ingredients:
- 2 eggs
- Cooking spray
- 1 teaspoon stevia
- 2 ounces cream cheese
- ½ teaspoon cinnamon, ground

Directions:
1. In your blender, mix eggs with cream cheese, stevia and cinnamon and blend well.
2. Heat up a pan with some cooking spray over medium high heat, pour ¼ of the batter, spread well, cook for 2 minutes, flip and cook for 1 minute more.
3. Transfer to a plate and repeat the action with the rest of the batter.
4. Serve them right away.

Enjoy!

Nutrition: calories 344, fat 23, fiber 12, carbs 3, protein 16

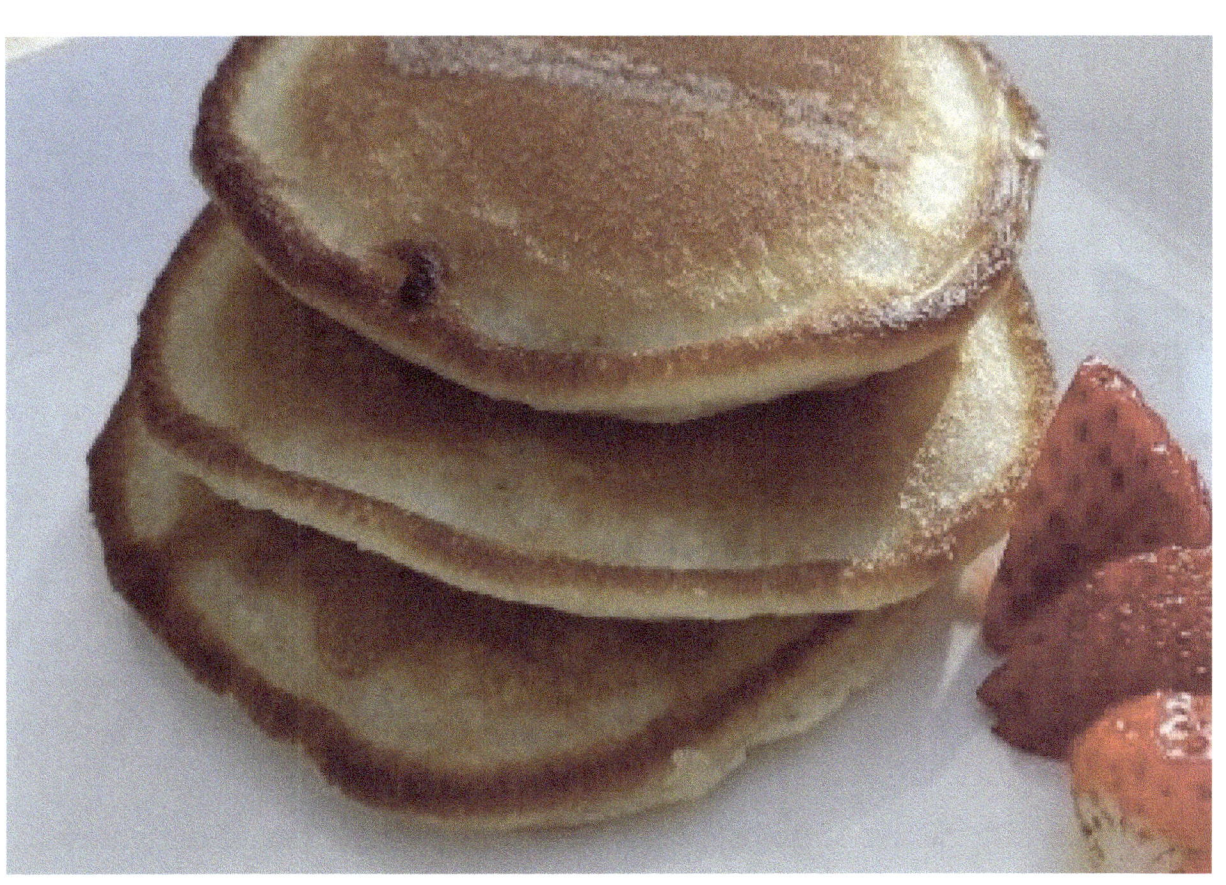

Pumpkin Pancakes

Preparation time: 10 minutes **Cooking time:** 15 minutes **Servings:** 6

Ingredients:
- 5 drops stevia
- 3 eggs
- ½ cup pumpkin puree
- 1 tablespoon swerve
- 1 teaspoon coconut oil
- 1 teaspoon vanilla extract
- 1 tablespoon chai masala
- 1 teaspoon baking powder
- 1 cup coconut cream
- 2 ounces hazelnut flour
- 2 ounces flax seeds, ground
- 1 ounce egg white protein

Directions:
1. In a bowl, mix flax seeds with hazelnut flour, egg white protein, baking powder and chai masala and stir.
2. In another bowl, mix coconut cream with vanilla extract, pumpkin puree, eggs, stevia and swerve and stir well.
3. Combine the 2 mixtures and stir well.
4. Heat up a pan with the oil over medium high heat, pour 1/6 of the batter, spread into a circle, cover, reduce heat to low, cook for 3 minutes on each side and transfer to a plate.
5. Repeat with the rest of the batter and serve your pumpkin pancakes right away. Enjoy!

Nutrition: calories 400, fat 23, fiber 4, carbs 5, protein 21

Delicious Waffles

Preparation time: 10 minutes **Cooking time:** 20 minutes **Servings:** 5

Ingredients:
- 2 teaspoon vanilla
- 4 tablespoons coconut flour
- 4 ounces ghee, melted
- 3 tablespoons stevia
- 1 teaspoon baking powder
- 5 eggs, separated
- 3 tablespoons almond milk

Directions:
1. In a bowl, whisk egg white using your mixer.
2. In another bowl mix flour with stevia, baking powder and egg yolks and whisk well.
3. Add vanilla, ghee and milk and stir well again.
4. Add egg white and stir gently everything.
5. Pour some of the mix into your waffle maker and cook until it's golden.
6. Repeat with the rest of the batter and serve your waffles right away.

Enjoy!

Nutrition: calories 240, fat 23, fiber 2, carbs 4, protein 7

The Perfect Smoothie

Preparation time: 5 minutes **Cooking time:** 0 minutes **Servings:** 1

Ingredients:
- 1 teaspoon whey protein
- 1 tablespoon psyllium seeds
- 1 tablespoon potato starch
- 10 almonds
- 2 cups spinach leaves
- 1 cup coconut milk
- 2 brazil nuts

Directions:
1. In your blender, mix spinach with brazil nuts, coconut milk and almonds and blend well.
2. Add green powder, whey protein, potato starch and psyllium seeds and blend well again.
3. Pour into a tall glass and consume for breakfast.

Enjoy!

Nutrition: calories 340, fat 30, fiber 7, carbs 7, protein 12

Breakfast Smoothie

Preparation time: 5 minutes **Cooking time:** 0 minutes **Servings:** 6

Ingredients:
- 1 cup cucumber, sliced
- 1 tablespoon swerve
- 1 tablespoon ginger, grated
- 4 cups water
- ½ avocado, pitted and peeled
- 1 cup lettuce leaves
- 1/3 cup pineapple, chopped
- ½ cup kiwi, peeled and sliced
- 2 tablespoons parsley leaves

Directions:
1. In your blender, mix water with lettuce leaves, pineapple, parsley, cucumber, ginger, kiwi, avocado and swerve and blend very well.
2. Pour into glasses and serve for a keto breakfast.

Enjoy!

Nutrition: calories 60, fat 2, fiber 3, carbs 3, protein 1

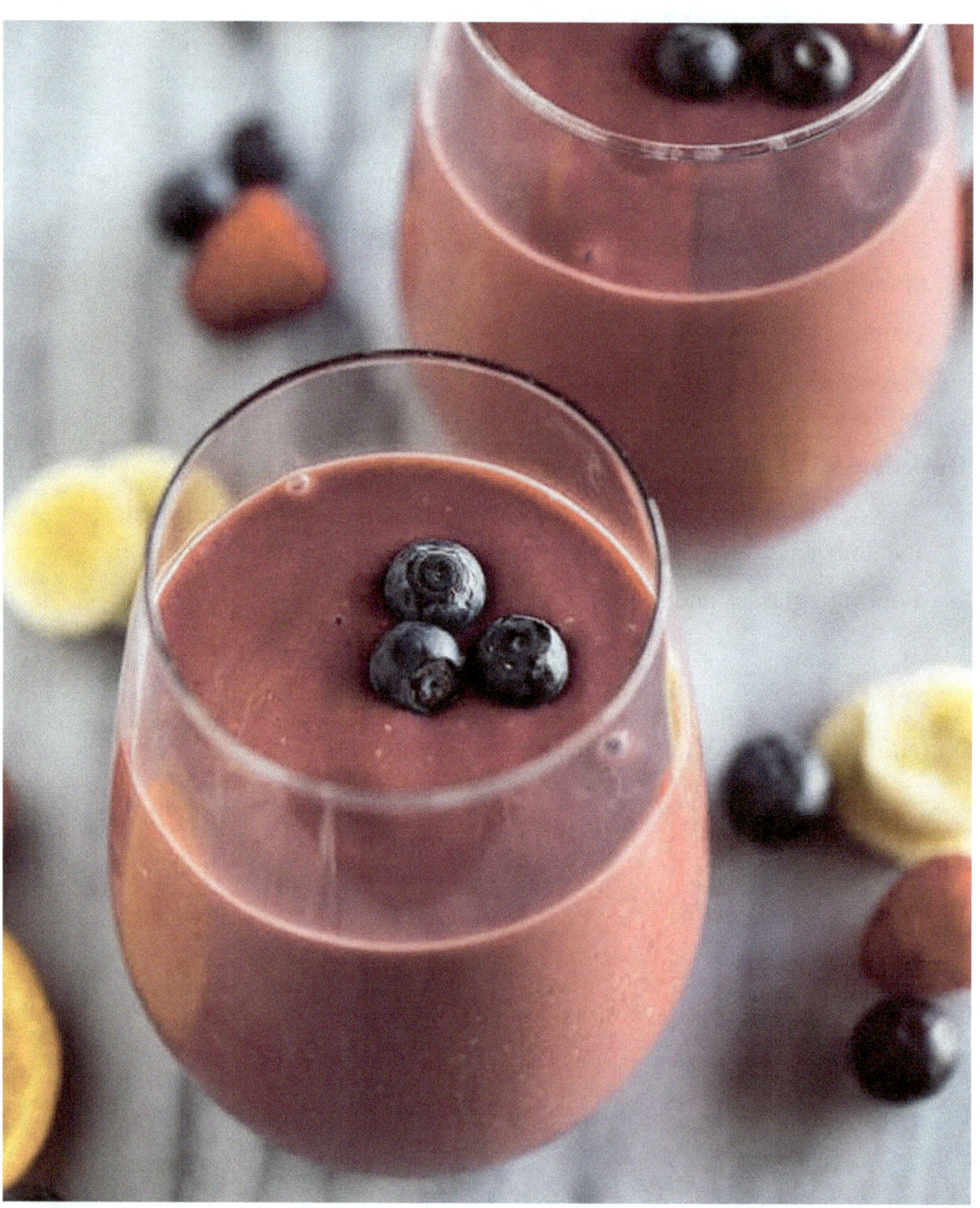

Chicken Quiche

Preparation time: 10 minutes **Cooking time:** 45 minutes **Servings:** 5

Ingredients:
- 1 teaspoon fennel seeds
- 1 teaspoon oregano, dried
- 1 pound chicken meat, ground
- 2 zucchinis, grated
- ½ cup heavy cream
- Salt and black pepper to the taste
- 2 tablespoons coconut oil
- 2 cups almond flour
- 7 eggs

Directions:
1. In your food processor, blend almond flour with a pinch of salt.
2. Add 1 egg and coconut oil and blend well.
3. Place dough in a greased pie pan and press well on the bottom.
4. Heat up a pan over medium heat, add chicken meat, brown for a couple of minutes, take off heat and leave aside.
5. In a bowl, mix 6 eggs with salt, pepper, oregano, cream and fennel seeds and whisk well.
6. Add chicken meat and stir again.
7. Pour this into pie crust, spread, introduce in the oven at 350 degrees F and bake for 40 minutes.
8. Leave the pie to cool down a bit before slicing and serving it for breakfast!

Enjoy!

Nutrition: calories 300, fat 23, fiber 3, carbs 4, protein 18

Chicken Omelet

Preparation time: 10 minutes **Cooking time:** 10 minutes **Servings:** 1

Ingredients:
- 2 eggs
- 1 small avocado, pitted, peeled and chopped
- Salt and black pepper to the taste
- 1 tomato, chopped
- 1 tablespoon homemade mayonnaise
- 2 bacon slices, cooked and crumbled
- 1 teaspoon mustard
- 1 ounce rotisserie chicken, shredded

Directions:
1. In a bowl, mix eggs with some salt and pepper and whisk gently.
2. Heat up a pan over medium heat, spray with some cooking oil, add eggs and cook your omelet for 5 minutes.
3. Add chicken, avocado, tomato, bacon, mayo and mustard on one half of the omelet.
4. Fold omelet, cover pan and cook for 5 minutes more.
5. Transfer to a plate and serve.

Enjoy!

Nutrition: calories 400, fat 32, fiber 6, carbs 4, protein 25

Easy Smoothie Bowl

Preparation time: 5 minutes **Cooking time:** 0 minutes **Servings: 1**

Ingredients:
- 4 walnuts
- 1 teaspoon chia seeds
- 1 tablespoon coconut ,shredded
- 4 raspberries
- 1 teaspoon protein powder
- ½ cup almond milk
- 1 cup spinach
- 1 tablespoon coconut oil
- 2 tablespoons heavy cream
- 2 ice cubes

Directions:
1. In your blender, mix milk with spinach, cream, ice, protein powder and coconut oil, blend well and transfer to a bowl.
2. Top your bowl with raspberries, coconut, walnuts and chia seeds and serve.

Enjoy!

Nutrition: calories 450, fat 34, fiber 4, carbs 4, protein 35

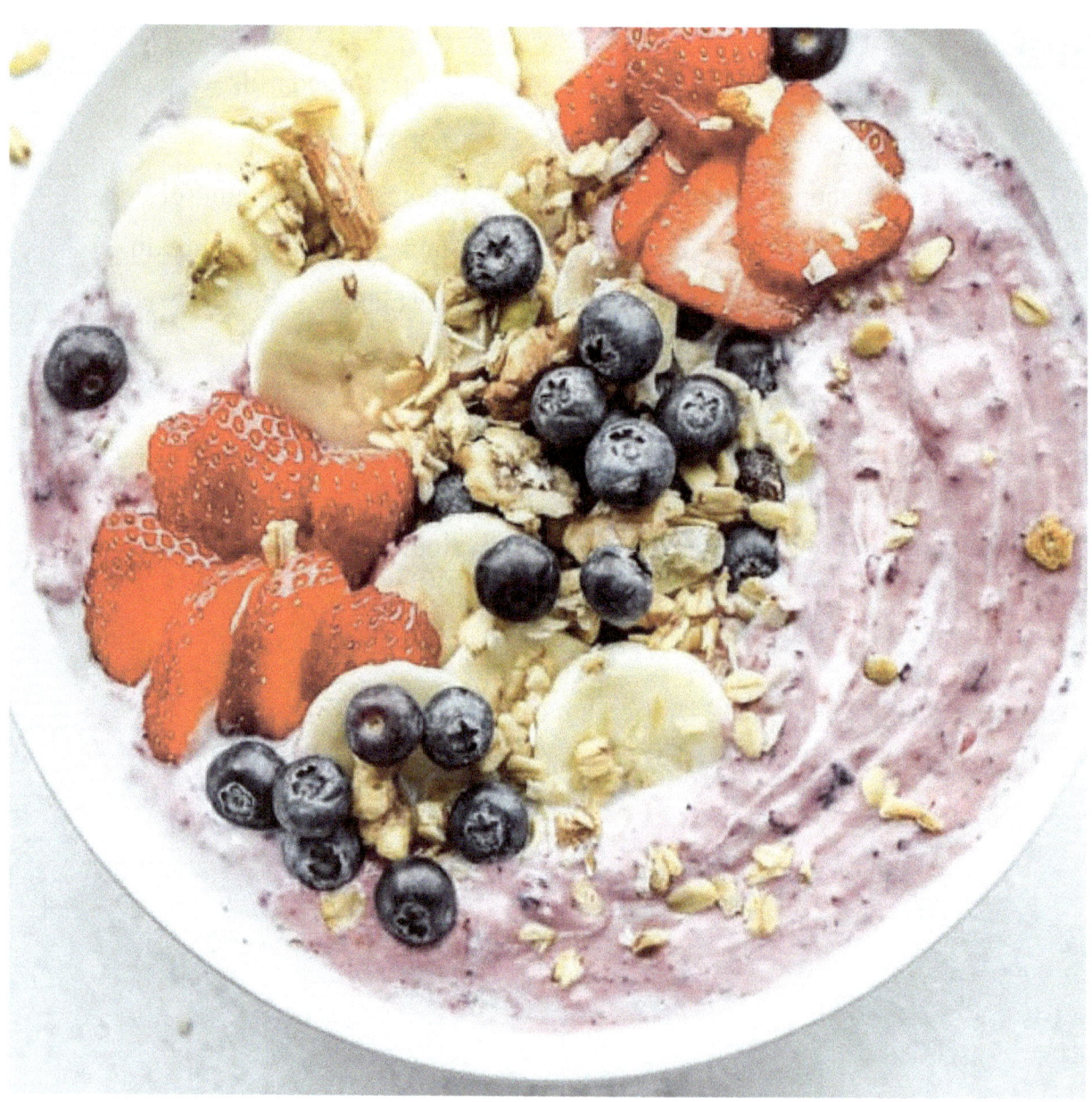

Breakfast Tuna Salad

Preparation time: 10 minutes **Cooking time:** 0 minutes **Servings: 4**

Ingredients:
- A pinch of chili flakes
- 1 tablespoon capers
- 8 tablespoons homemade mayonnaise
- 4 leeks, finely chopped
- Salt and black pepper to the taste
- 2 tablespoons sour cream
- 12 ounces tuna in olive oil

Directions:
1. In a salad bowl, mix tuna with capers, salt, pepper, leeks, chili flakes, sour cream and mayo.
2. Stir well and serve with some crispy bread.

Enjoy!

Nutrition: calories 160, fat 2, fiber 1, carbs 2, protein 6

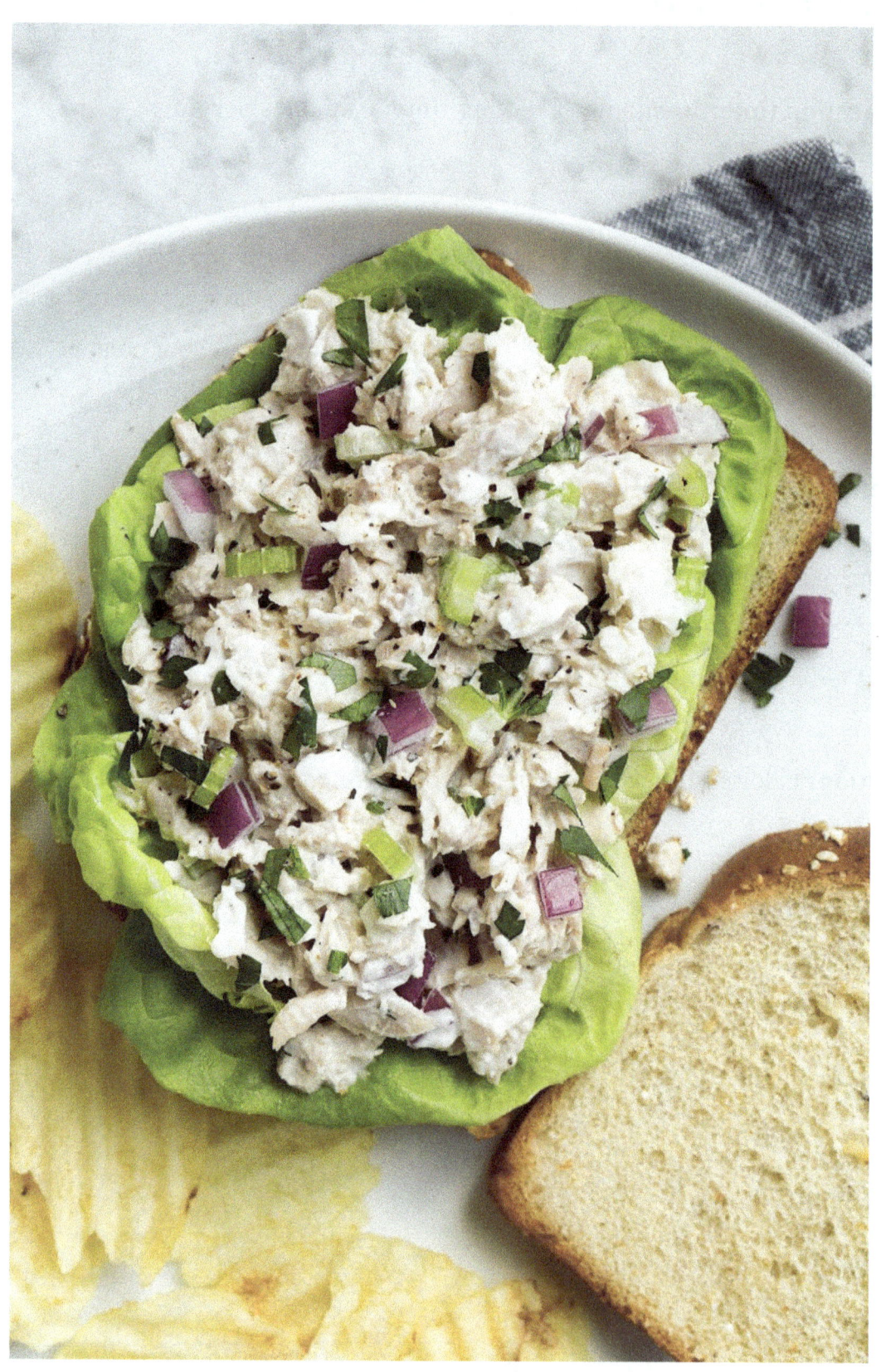

Naan Bread And Butter

Preparation time: 10 minutes **Cooking time:** 10 minutes **Servings:** 6

Ingredients:
- Salt to the taste
- 2 cups hot water
- 2 tablespoons psyllium powder
- ½ teaspoon baking powder
- 7 tablespoons coconut oil
- ¾ cup coconut flour
- 3.5 ounces ghee
- Some coconut oil for frying
- 2 garlic cloves, minced

Directions:
1. In a bowl, mix coconut flour with baking powder, salt and psyllium powder and stir.
2. Add 7 tablespoons coconut oil and the hot water and start kneading your dough.
3. Leave aside for 5 minutes, divide into 6 balls and flatten them on a working surface.
4. Heat up a pan with some coconut oil over medium high heat, add naan breads to the pan, fry them until they are golden and transfer them to a plate.
5. Heat up a pan with the ghee over medium high heat, add garlic, salt and pepper, stir and cook for 2 minutes.
6. Brush naan breads with this mix and pour the rest into a bowl.
7. Serve in the morning.

Enjoy!

Nutrition: calories 140, fat 9, fiber 2, carbs 3, protein 4

Ketogenic Recipes For Lunch

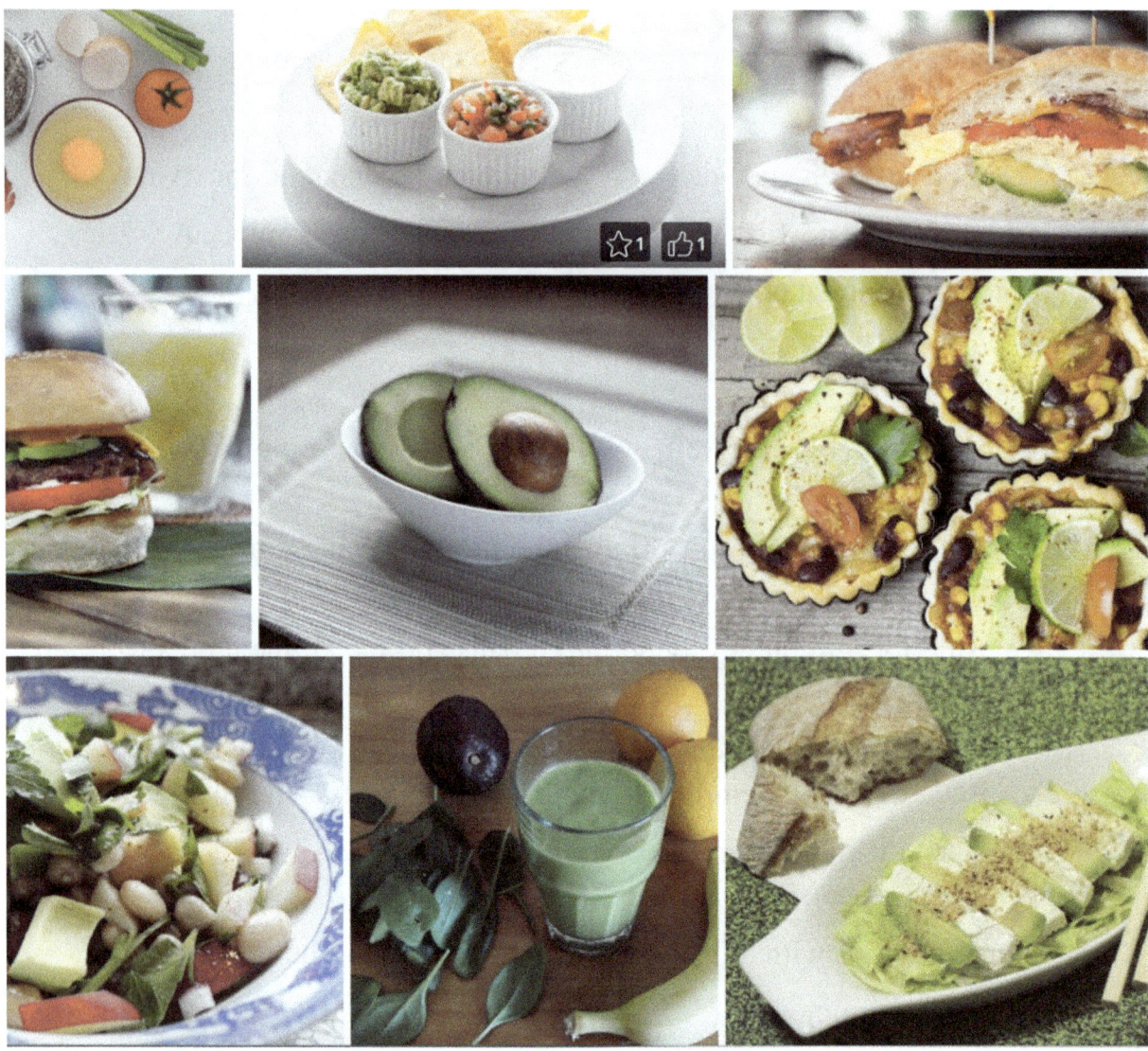

Caesar Salad

Preparation time: 10 minutes **Cooking time:** 0 minutes **Servings:** 2

Ingredients:
- 1 cup bacon, cooked and crumbled
- 1 chicken breast, grilled and shredded
- 3 tablespoons creamy Caesar dressing
- Salt and black pepper to the taste
- 1 avocado, pitted, peeled and sliced

Directions:
1. In a salad bowl, mix avocado with bacon and chicken breast and stir.
2. Add Caesar dressing, salt and pepper, toss to coat, divide into 2 bowls and serve.

Enjoy!

Nutrition: calories 334, fat 23, fiber 4, carbs 3, protein 18

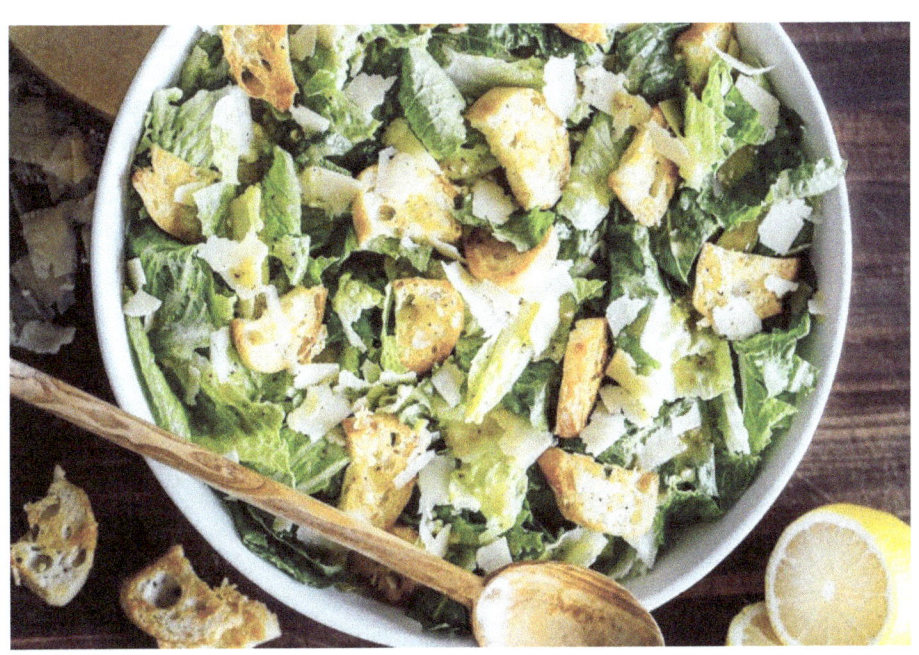

Pizza

Preparation time: 10 minutes **Cooking time:** 7 minutes **Servings:** 4

Ingredients:
- 1 cup pizza cheese mix, shredded
- 1 tablespoon olive oil
- 1/3 cup broccoli florets, steamed
- Some asiago cheese, shaved for serving
- 2 tablespoons ghee
- 1 cup mozzarella cheese, shredded
- 1 teaspoon garlic, minced
- Salt and black pepper to the taste
- ¼ cup mascarpone cheese
- 1 tablespoon heavy cream

Directions:
1. Heat up a pan with the oil over medium heat, add pizza cheese mix and spread into a circle.
2. Add mozzarella cheese and also spread into a circle.
3. Cook everything for 5 minutes and transfer to a plate.
4. Heat up the pan with the ghee over medium heat, add mascarpone cheese, cream, salt, pepper, lemon pepper and garlic, stir and cook for 5 minutes.
5. Drizzle half of this mix over cheese crust.
6. Add broccoli florets to the pan with the rest of the mascarpone mix, stir and cook for 1 minute.
7. Add this on top of the pizza, sprinkle asiago cheese at the end and serve.

Enjoy!

Nutrition: calories 250, fat 15, fiber 1, carbs 3, protein 10

Chocolate Protein Pancakes

Preparation Time: 10 minutes **Cooking Time:** 15 minutes **Servings:** 12

Ingredients:
- ½ cup of almond flour, blanched
- ½ cup of whey protein powder
- 1 tsp. of baking powder
- 1/8 tsp. of sea salt
- 3 tbsp. of erythritol sweetener
- 1 tsp. of vanilla extract, unsweetened
- 3 tbsp. of cocoa powder, organic, unsweetened
- 4 Eggs, pastured
- 2 tbsp. of avocado oil
- 1/3 cup of almond milk, unsweetened

Kitchen Equipment:
- immersion blender
- medium skillet pan
- freezer bag
- parchment paper
- microwave or oven

Directions:

1. Transfer all the ingredients in a large mixing bowl, beat using an immersion blender or until well combined and then let the mixture stand for 5 minutes.

2. Then take a medium skillet pan, place it over medium-low heat, grease it with avocado oil and pour in prepared pancake batter in small circles of about 3-inches diameter.

3. Cover the skillet pan with lid, let the pancakes cook for 3 minutes or until bubbles form on top, then flip them and continue cooking for 1 to 2 minutes or until nicely golden brown.

4. Cook remaining pancakes, in the same manner, you will end up with 12 pancakes, and then let them cool at room temperature.

5. Place cooled pancakes in a freezer bag, with parchment sheet between them and store them in the refrigerator for 5 to 7 days.

6. When ready to serve, microwave pancakes for 30 seconds to 1 minute or bake in the oven for 5 minutes until thoroughly heated.

Nutrition: Calories: 237 **Fat:** 20g **Protein:** 11g

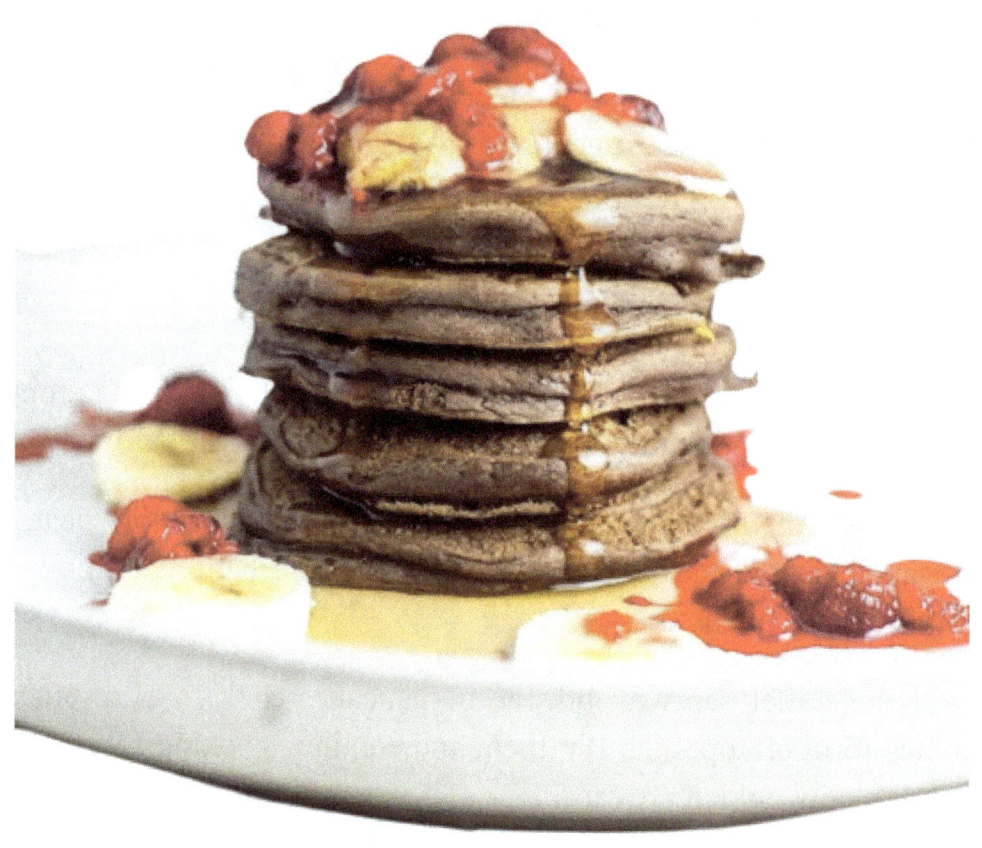

Pizza Rolls

Preparation time: 10 minutes **Cooking time:** 30 minutes **Servings:** 6

Ingredients:
- 2 cup mozzarella cheese, shredded
- 1 teaspoon pizza seasoning
- ¼ cup mixed red and green bell peppers, chopped
- 2 tablespoons onion, chopped
- Salt and black pepper to the taste
- 1 tomato, chopped
- ¼ cup pizza sauce
- ½ cup sausage, crumbled and cooked

Directions:
1. Spread mozzarella cheese on a lined and lightly greased baking sheet, sprinkle pizza seasoning on top, introduce in the oven at 400 degrees F and bake for 20 minutes.
2. 2. Take your pizza crust out of the oven, spread sausage, onion, bell peppers and tomatoes all over and drizzle the tomato sauce at the end.
3. 3. Introduce in the oven again and bake for 10 minutes more.
4. 4. Take pizza out of the oven, leave aside for a couple of minutes, slice into 6 pieces, roll each piece and serve for lunch!

Enjoy!

Nutrition: calories 117, fat 7, fiber 1, carbs 2, protein 11

Stuffed Peppers

Preparation time: 10 minutes **Cooking time:** 40 minutes **Servings:** 4

Ingredients:
- 1 tablespoon ghee
- 4 big banana peppers, tops cut off, seeds removed and cut into halves lengthwise
- Some marinara sauce
- A drizzle of olive oil
- 1 pound sweet sausage, chopped
- 3 tablespoons yellow onions, chopped
- ½ teaspoon herbs de Provence
- Salt and black pepper to the taste

Directions:
1. Season banana peppers with salt and pepper, drizzle the oil, rub well and bake in the oven at 350 degrees F for 20 minutes.
2. 2. Meanwhile, heat up a pan over medium heat, add sausage pieces, stir and cook for 5 minutes.
3. 3. Add onion, herbs de Provence, salt, pepper and ghee, stir well and cook for 5 minutes.
4. 4. Take peppers out of the oven, fill them with the sausage mix, place them in an oven-proof dish, drizzle marinara sauce over them, introduce in the oven again and bake for 10 minutes more.
5. 5. Serve hot.

Enjoy!

Nutrition: calories 320, fat 8, fiber 4, carbs 3, protein 10

Burgers

Preparation time: 10 minutes **Cooking time:** 25 minutes **Servings:** 8

Ingredients:
- 2 tablespoons olive oil
- 1 pound brisket, ground
- 1 yellow onion, chopped
- 1 tablespoon water
- 1 tablespoon Italian seasoning
- 2 tablespoons mayonnaise
- 1 tablespoon ghee
- 1 tablespoon garlic, minced
- Salt and black pepper to the taste
- 8 butter slices
- 1 pound beef, ground

Directions:
1. In a bowl, mix brisket with beef, salt, pepper, Italian seasoning, garlic and mayo and stir well.
2. Shape 8 patties and make a pocket in each.
3. Stuff each burger with a butter slice and seal.
4. Heat up a pan with the olive oil over medium heat, add onions, stir and cook for 2 minutes.
5. Add the water, stir and gather them in the corner of the pan.
6. Place burgers in the pan with the onions and cook them over medium-low heat for 10 minutes.
7. Flip them, add the ghee and cook them for 10 minutes more.
8. 8. Divide burgers on buns and serve them with caramelized onions on top.

Enjoy!

Nutrition: calories 180, fat 8, fiber 1, carbs 4, protein 20

Avocado Egg Bake

Preparation Time: 5 minutes **Cooking Time:** 15 minutes **Servings:** 1

Ingredients:

- 1 tbsp. of fresh parsley, chopped
- 1 avocado, cut in half and the pits removed
- Salt to taste
- Ground black pepper to your preferred taste
- 2 eggs
- ¼ cup of cheddar cheese shredded

Kitchen Equipment:

- oven
- baking sheet

Directions:

1. Preheat the oven to 425 degrees F.
2. The next thing to do is scoop some avocado from the pitted area.
3. Place both halves of the avocado on a baking sheet and break an egg onto each avocado.
4. Let it bake in the oven for about 20 minutes. Only stop baking when you are sure the eggs are cooked.
5. Add salt and pepper to season the avocado egg, and garnish with cheddar cheese and parsley.

Nutrition: Calories: 605 - **Protein:** 25.3g - **Fat:** 50.9g

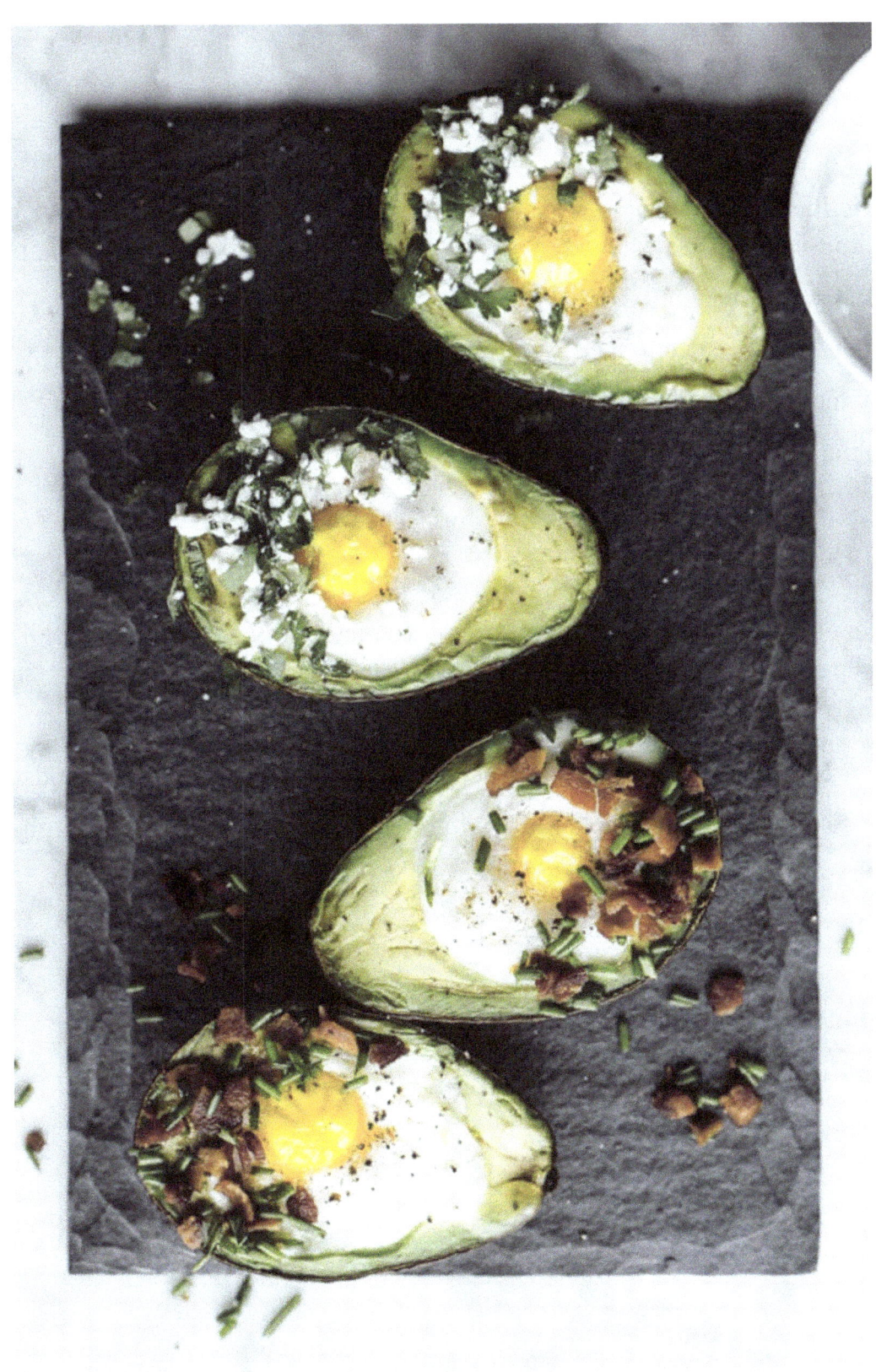

Zucchini Dish

Preparation time: 10 minutes **Cooking time:** 5 minutes **Servings:** 1

Ingredients:
- ¼ cup asiago cheese, shaved
- ¼ cup parmesan, grated
- 1 tablespoon basil, chopped
- Salt and black pepper to the taste
- 1 tablespoon garlic, minced
- 1 tablespoon red bell pepper, chopped
- 2 cups zucchini, cut with a spiralizer
- 1 teaspoon red pepper flakes
- 1 tablespoon olive oil
- 3 tablespoons ghee

Directions:
1. Heat up a pan with the oil and ghee over medium heat, add garlic, bell pepper and pepper flakes, stir and cook for 1 minute.
2. 2. Add zucchini noodles, stir and cook for 2 minutes more.
3. 3. Add basil, parmesan, salt and pepper, stir and cook for a few seconds more.
4. 4. Take off heat, transfer to a bowl and serve for lunch with asiago cheese on top.

Enjoy!

Nutrition: calories 140, fat 3, fiber 1, carbs 1.3, protein 5

Turkey-Pepper Mix

Preparation Time: 20 minutes **Cooking Time:** 0 minute **Servings:** 1

Ingredients:
- 1-pound of turkey tenderloin (cut in thin steaks)
- 1 tsp. of salt, divided)
- 2 tbsp. of extra-virgin olive oil (divided)
- ½ sweet onion (sliced)
- 1 red bell pepper (cut into strips)
- 1 yellow bell pepper (cut into strips)
- ½ tsp. of Italian seasoning
- ¼ tsp. of ground black pepper
- 2 tsp. of red wine vinegar
- 1 14-ounces can of crushed tomatoes, roasted
- Fresh parsley
- Basil

Kitchen Equipment:
- pan

Directions:
1. Sprinkle ½ tsp. of salt on your turkey.
2. Drizzle 1 tablespoon of oil into the pan and heat it.
3. Add the turkey steaks and cook for 1–3 minutes per side. Set aside.
4. Put the onion, bell peppers, and the remaining salt to the pan and cook for 7 minutes, stirring all the time.
5. Sprinkle with Italian seasoning and add black pepper.
6. Cook for 30 seconds.
7. Add the tomatoes and vinegar and fry the mix for about 20 seconds.
8. Place the turkey back to the pan and pour the sauce over it.

9. Simmer for 2–3 minutes.

10. Top with chopped parsley and basil.

Nutrition: Carbohydrates: 11g **Protein:** 30g **Calories:** 230

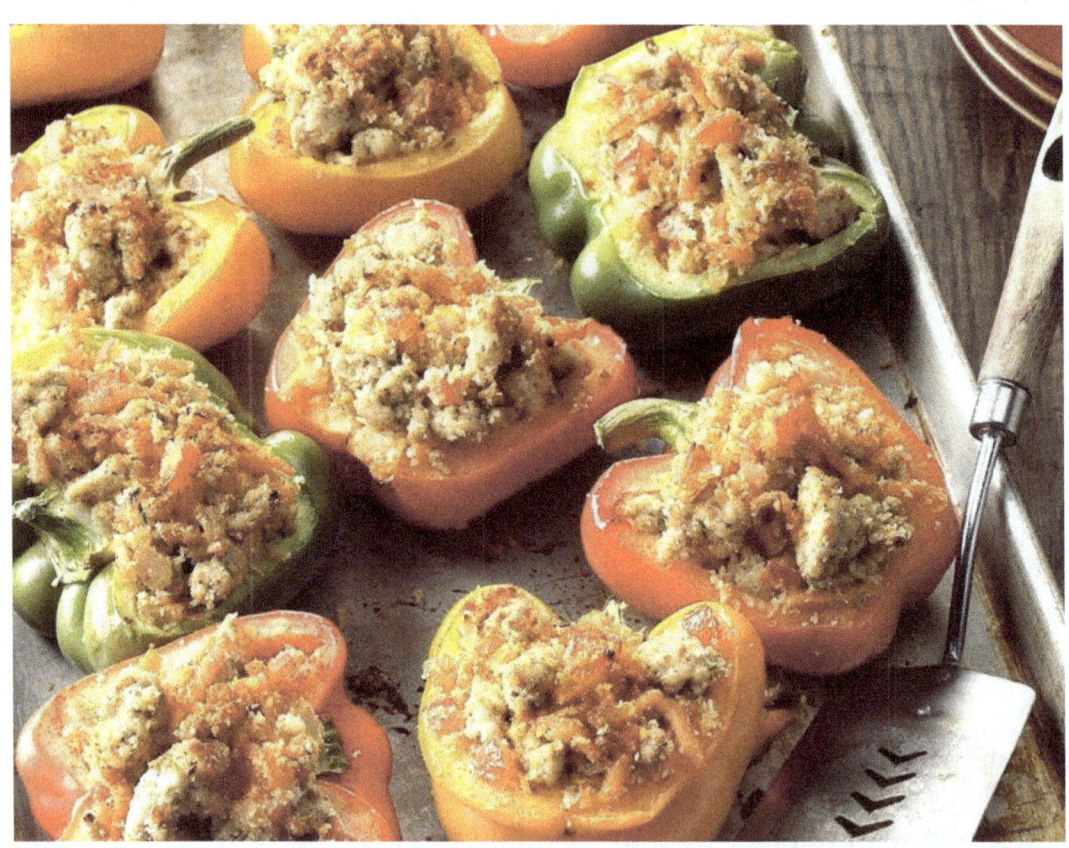

Ingredient Zucchini Lasagna

Preparation Time: 10 minutes **Cooking Time:** 1 hour 20 minutes **Servings:** 9

Ingredients:

For ricotta:
- 3 cups of raw macadamia nuts
- 2 tbsp. of nutritional yeast
- 2 tsp. of dried oregano
- 1 tsp. of sea salt
- 1/2 cup of water
- 1/4 cup of vegan parmesan cheese
- 1/2 cup of fresh basil, chopped
- 1 medium lemon, juiced
- Black pepper to taste

Sauce:
- 1 28-oz jar favorite marinara sauce
- 3 medium zucchini squash thinly sliced

Kitchen Equipment:
- mandolin
- oven
- food processor
- pan
- aluminum foil

Directions:

1. Prepare the oven to 375 degrees Fahrenheit.
2. Put macadamia nuts to a food processor.
3. Add the remaining ingredients and continue to puree the mixture. You need to create a fine paste.
4. Taste and adjust the seasonings depending on your personal preferences.
5. Pour 1 cup of marinara sauce in a baking dish.

6. Start creating the lasagna layers using thinly sliced zucchini
7. Scoop small amounts of ricotta mixture on the zucchini and spread it into a thin layer.
8. Continue the layering until you've run out of zucchini or space for it.
9. Sprinkle parmesan cheese on the topmost layer.
10. Wrap it with foil then bake for 45 minutes.
11. Remove the foil and bake for 15 minutes more.
12. Allow it to cool for 15 minutes before serving.
13. Serve immediately.
14. The lasagna will keep for 3 days in the fridge.

Nutrition: Calories: 338 **Fat:** 34g **Carbohydrates:** 10g

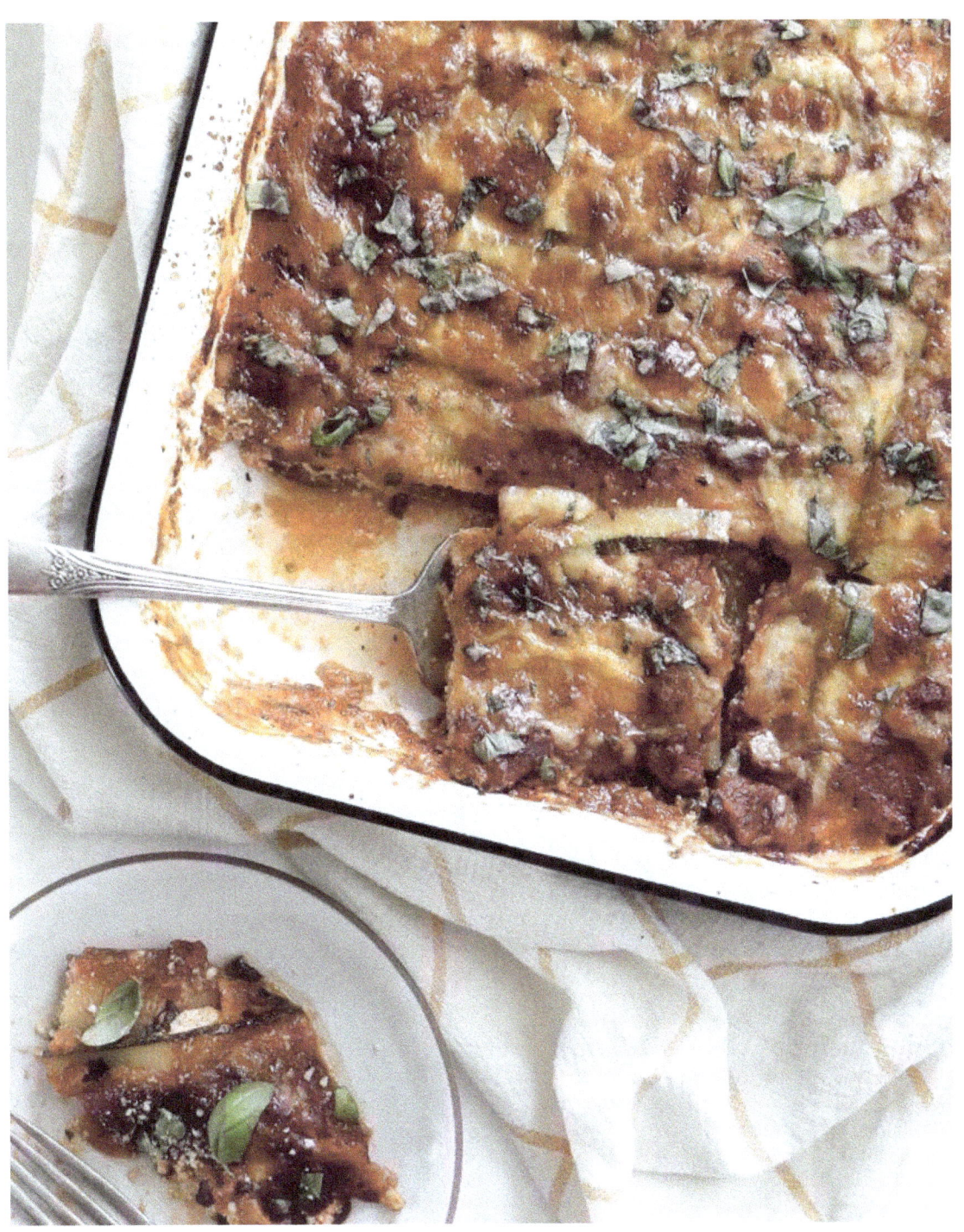

Salad

Preparation time: 10 minutes **Cooking time:** 0 minutes **Servings:** 3

Ingredients:

- 1/3 cup mayonnaise
- A pinch of granulated garlic
- 1 teaspoon mustard
- ½ tablespoons dill relish
- 1 green onion, chopped
- Salt and black pepper to the taste
- 2 tablespoons parsley, chopped
- 5 ounces chicken breast, roasted and chopped
- 1 egg, hard-boiled, peeled and chopped
- 1 celery rib, chopped

Directions:

1. In your food processor, mix parsley with onion and celery and pulse well.
2. Transfer these to a bowl and leave aside for now.
3. Put chicken meat in your food processor, blend well and add to the bowl with the veggies.
4. Add egg pieces, salt and pepper and stir.
5. Also add mustard, mayo, dill relish and granulated garlic, toss to coat and serve right away.

Enjoy!

Nutrition: calories 283, fat 23, fiber 5, carbs 3, protein 12

Cold Avocado and Crab Soup

Preparation Time: 15 minutes **Cooking Time:** 0 minute **Servings:** 6

Ingredients:
- ½ onion, diced
- ½ cup of fresh cilantro, roughly chopped
- 1 cup of watercress
- 1 cup of heavy whipping cream
- 1 English cucumber, cut into chunks
- 2 avocados, diced
- 2 cups of coconut water
- 2 teaspoons of ground cumin
- Juice of 1 lime
- Salt and black pepper, to taste
- 1 pound (454 g) of cooked crab meat

Kitchen Equipment:
- blender
- large bowl

Directions:

1. Incorporate all the ingredients, except for the crab meat, in a blender.
2. Process until smooth.
3. Pour the soup in a large bowl.
4. Add the crab meat into the soup and serve immediately

Nutrition: Calories: 298 - **Total fat:** 23.1g - **Fiber:** 4.1g

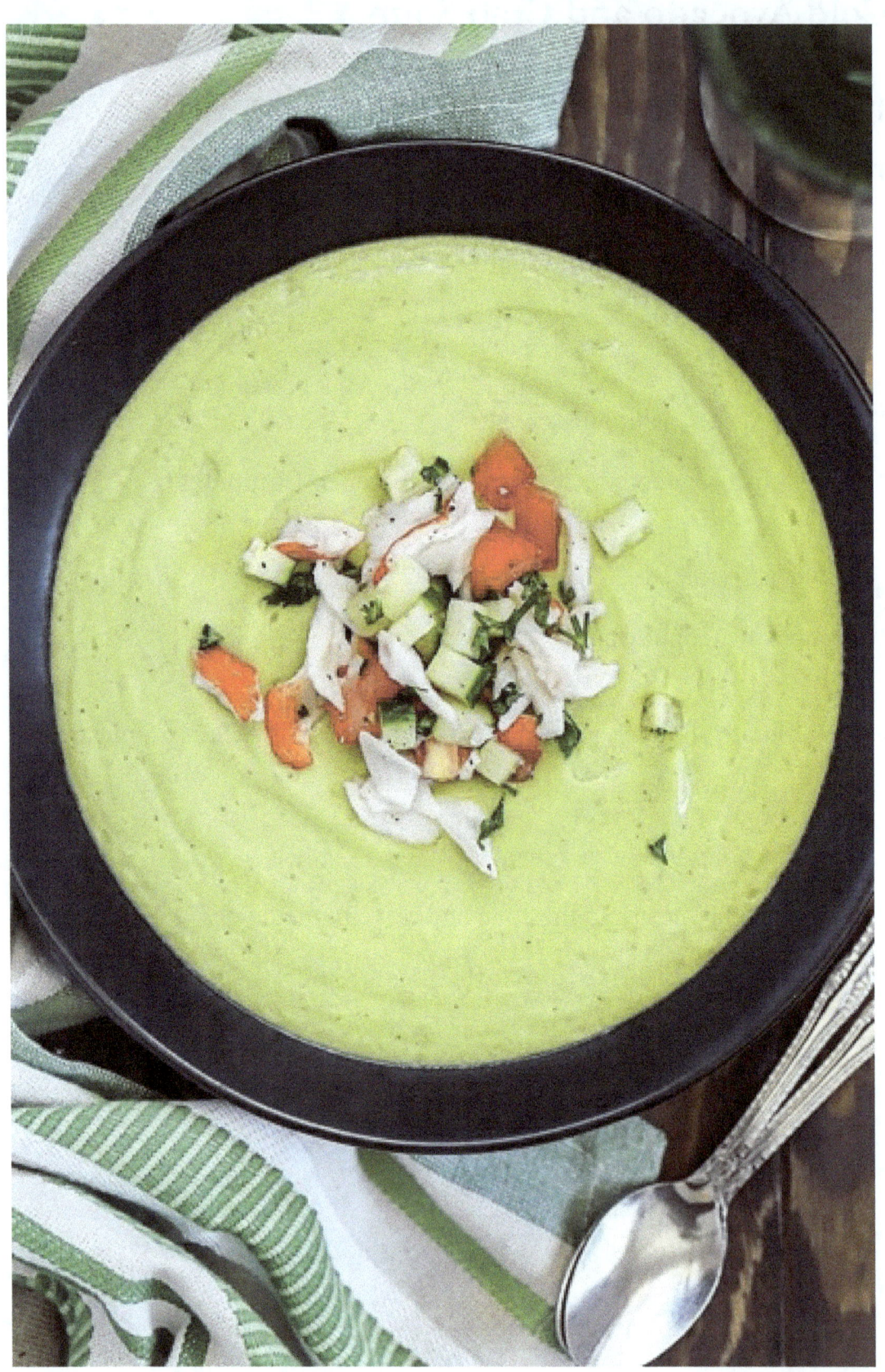

Balsamic Chicken

Preparation Time: 10 minutes **Cooking Time:** 60 minutes **Servings:** 4

Ingredients:
- 4 pcs. of chicken breast
- 2 tbsp. of grass-fed butter
- A dash salt
- 4 roasted garlic cloves
- 2 cups of mushrooms
- 1 tsp. of thyme
- 1 tbsp. of chives
- 1 tsp. of red pepper flakes
- ¼ cup of balsamic vinegar
- ½ cup of water
- ¼ cup of onions

Kitchen Equipment:
- stove
- baking sheet
- skillet

Directions:

1. Prepare the stove to 350 and getting out your baking sheet.

2. As the stove warms up, take out your skillet and begin heating the butter in it. Once melted, mix in the chicken pieces and season with your pepper and salt. When the meat is seasoned to your taste, grill each side of the chicken for 3 or 4 minutes. Once it's cooked thoroughly, transfer it onto your baking sheet, and cook in your heated stove for additional 25 minutes.

3. While the chicken cooks, melt some more butter in your heated pan. Once melted, sauté mushrooms and onions. Mix in the roasted garlic, thyme, red pepper flakes, and the balsamic vinegar. After these ingredients have cooked for a minute, pour in the water and stir until the liquid begins to reduce.

4. Pour the mixture over your chicken and serve the dish hot. If you would like, you can serve with fresh parsley or chopped chives for some nice additional flavors.

Nutrition: Fats: 15g **Carbs:** 8g **Proteins:** 30g

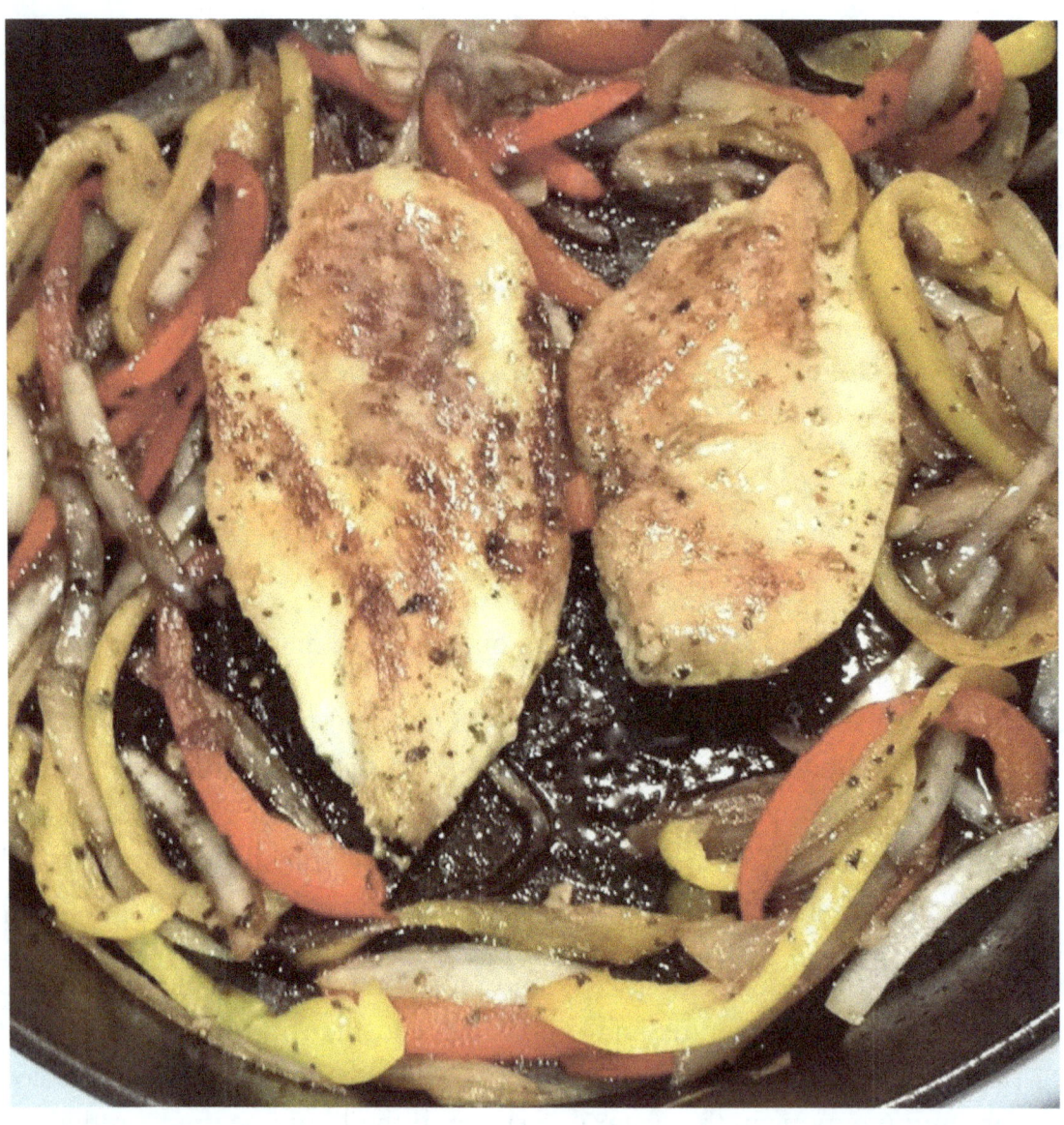

Steak Salad

Preparation time: 10 minutes **Cooking time:** 20 minutes **Servings:**

Ingredients:
- 1 teaspoon onion powder
- 1 orange bell pepper, sliced
- 1 teaspoon Italian seasoning
- 1 avocado, pitted, peeled and sliced
- 3 ounces sun-dried tomatoes, chopped
- 1 yellow bell pepper, sliced
- 1 and ½ pound steak, thinly sliced
- 3 tablespoons avocado oil
- 6 ounces sweet onion, chopped
- Salt and black pepper to the taste
- ¼ cup balsamic vinegar
- 4 1 teaspoon red pepper flakes
- 4 ounces mushrooms, sliced
- 2 garlic cloves, minced
- 1 lettuce head, chopped

Directions:
1. In a bowl, mix steak pieces with some salt, pepper and balsamic vinegar, toss to coat and leave aside for now.
2. 2. Heat up a pan with the avocado oil over medium-low heat, add mushrooms, garlic, salt, pepper and onion, stir and cook for 20 minutes.
3. 3. In a bowl, mix lettuce leaves with orange and yellow bell pepper, sun dried tomatoes and avocado and stirred.
4. 4. Season steak pieces with onion powder, pepper flakes and Italian seasoning.
5. 5. Place steak pieces in a broiling pan, introduce in preheated broiler and cook for 5 minutes.
6. 6. Divide steak pieces on plates, add lettuce and avocado salad on the side and top everything with onion and mushroom mix.

Enjoy!

Nutrition: calories 435, fat 23, fiber 7, carbs 10, protein 35

Spinach and Red Pepper Frittata

Preparation Time: 5 minutes **Cooking Time:** 22 minutes **Servings:** 8

Ingredients:
- 8 eggs
- 1/3 cup of heavy whipping cream
- ½ cup of shredded cheddar cheese
- ¼ cup of diced red bell pepper
- ¼ cup of minced red onion
- ½ cup of chopped spinach
- 1 tsp. of sea salt
- 1 tsp. of red chili powder
- 1/8 tsp. of Ground black pepper
- 1 cup of water
- 1 avocado (peeled, pitted, sliced)
- ½ cup of sour cream

Kitchen Equipment:
- 7-inch baking dish
- instant pot
- trivet stand

Directions:
1. Break eggs in a bowl, add cream and whisk until beaten and fluffy.
2. Add remaining ingredients, except for water, avocado and sour cream, stir well until incorporated and then pour the mixture in a 7-inch baking dish greased with avocado oil.
3. Switch on the instant pot, pour water in it, insert a trivet stand and place baking dish on it.
4. Seal the instant pot, then click the 'manual' button, press '+/-' to adjust the cooking time to 12 minutes and press high-pressure setting; when the pressure starts, the timer will start.
5. When the instant pot rings, select the 'keep warm' button, let the pressure release naturally for 10 minutes. Then slowly open the pot.
6. Take out the baking dish and take out the frittata by inverting the dish onto a plate, and cut into slices.
7. Serve straight away.

Nutrition: Calories: 218 - **Fat:** 17.6g - **Protein:** 9.4g

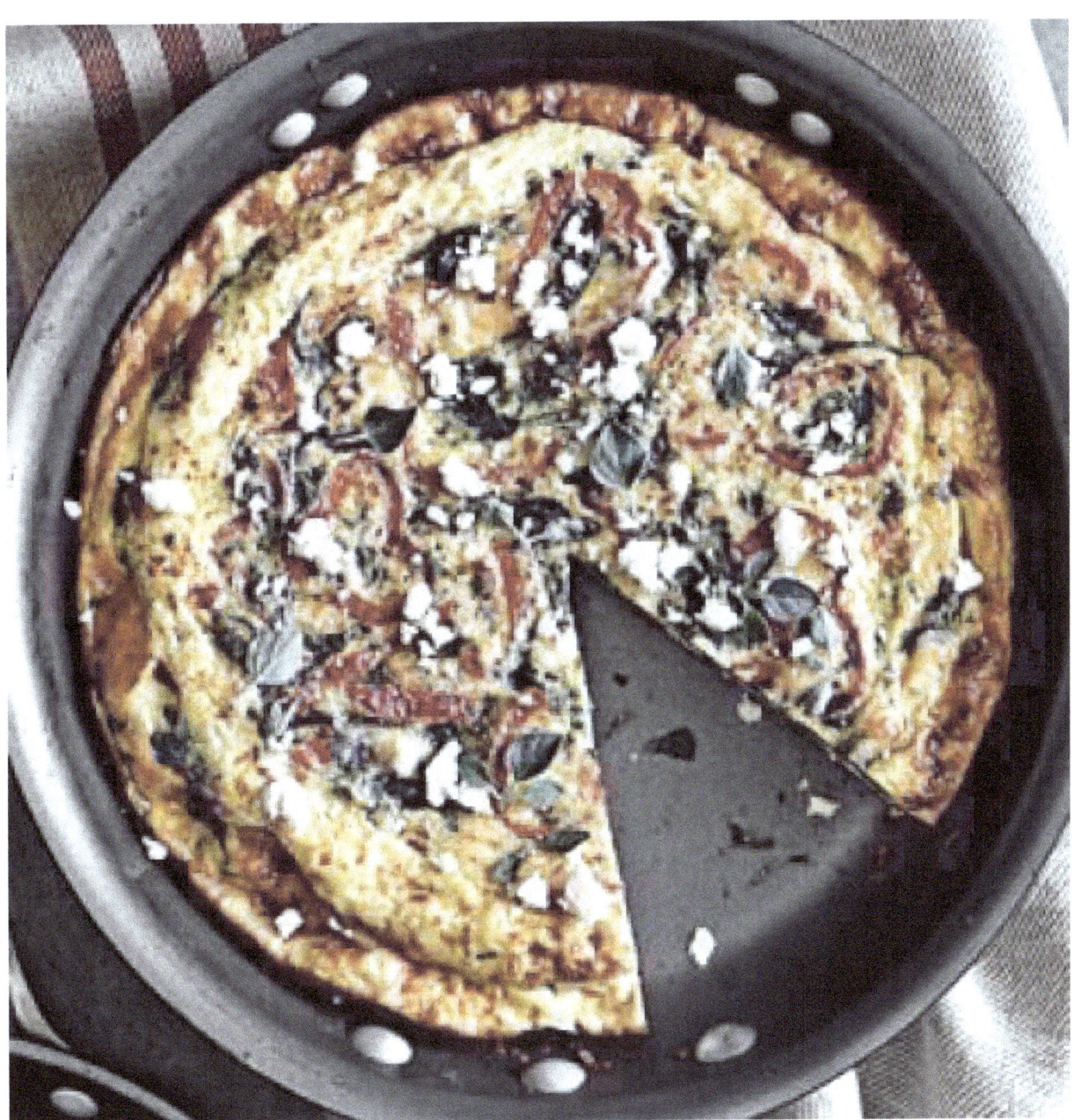

Stuffed Avocado

Preparation time: 10 minutes **Cooking time:** 0 minutes **Servings:** 1

Ingredients:
- 1 tablespoon lemon juice
- Salt and black pepper to the taste
- 1 tablespoon mayonnaise
- 1 spring onion, chopped
- ¼ teaspoon turmeric powder
- 4 ounces canned sardines, drained
- 1 avocado

Directions:
1. Cut avocado in halves, scoop flesh and put in a bowl.
2. Mash with a fork and mix with sardines.
3. Mash again with your fork and mix with onion, lemon juice, turmeric powder, salt, pepper and mayo.
4. Stir everything and divide into avocado halves.
5. Serve for lunch right away.

Enjoy!

Nutrition: calories 230, fat 34, fiber 12, carbs 5, protein 27

Chicken Pan with Veggies and Pesto

Preparation Time: 10 minutes **Cooking Time:** 20 minutes **Servings:** 4

Ingredients:
- 2 tbsp. of olive oil
- 1-pound of chicken thighs (boneless, skinless, sliced into strips)
- ¾ cup of oil-packed sun-dried tomatoes (chopped)
- 1-pound of asparagus ends
- ¼ cup of basil pesto
- 1 cup of cherry tomatoes (red and yellow, halved)
- Salt (to taste)

Kitchen Equipment:
- frying pan
- skillet

Directions:
1. Cook olive oil in a frying pan over medium-high heat.
2. Put salt on the chicken slices and then put into a skillet, add the sun-dried tomatoes and fry for 5–10 minutes.
3. Remove the chicken slices and season with salt.
4. Add asparagus to the skillet.
5. Cook for additional 5–10 minutes.
6. Transfer the chicken back in the skillet, pour in the pesto and whisk.
7. Fry for 1–2 minutes.
8. Remove from the heat.
9. Add the halved cherry tomatoes and pesto.
10. Stir well and serve.

Nutrition: Carbohydrates: 12g - **Protein:** 2g - **Calories:** 423

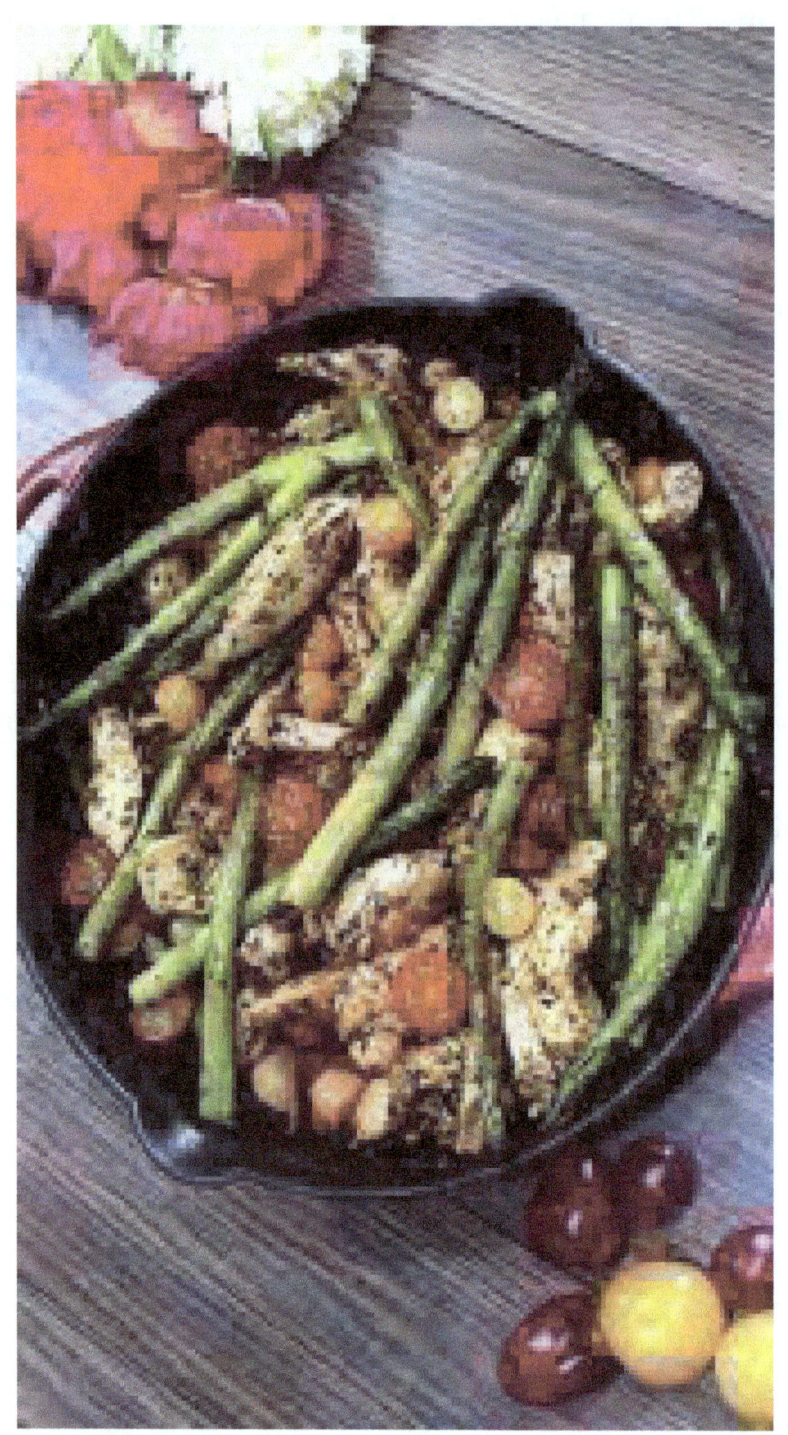

Crab Cakes

Preparation time: 10 minutes **Cooking time:** 12 minutes **Servings:** 6

Ingredients:
- 1 pound crabmeat
- 2 tablespoons olive oil
- 1 egg
- ½ cup mayonnaise
- ½ teaspoon mustard powder
- ¼ cup parsley, chopped
- 2 green onions, chopped
- Salt and black pepper to the taste
- ¼ cup cilantro, chopped
- 1 teaspoon lemon juice
- 1 teaspoon jalapeno pepper, minced
- 1 teaspoon Worcestershire sauce
- 1 teaspoon old bay seasoning

Directions:
1. In a large bowl mix crab meat with salt, pepper, parsley, green onions, cilantro, jalapeno, lemon juice, old bay seasoning, mustard powder and Worcestershire sauce and stir very well.
2. In another bowl mix egg wit mayo and whisk.
3. Add this to crabmeat mix and stir everything.
4. Shape 6 patties from this mix and place them on a plate.
5. Heat up a pan with the oil over medium high heat, add 3 crab cakes, cook for 3 minutes, flip, cook them for 3 minutes more and transfer to paper towels.
6. 6. Repeat with the other 3 crab cakes, drain excess grease and serve for lunch.

Enjoy!

Nutrition: calories 254, fat 17, fiber 1, carbs 1, protein 20

Frittata

Preparation Time: 5 minutes **Cooking Time:** 17 minutes **Servings:** 1

Ingredients:
- 5oz of bacon slices (pastured, diced)
- ½ medium red onion (peeled, diced)
- ½ red bell pepper (cored, diced)
- ¼ tsp. of salt
- 1 tsp. of ground black pepper
- 3 tbsp. of avocado oil
- ¼ cup and 2 tbsp. of grated parmesan cheese (full-fat)
- 6 eggs (pastured)

Kitchen Equipment:
- 8-inch skillet pan
- broiler
- microwave

Directions:
1. Take an 8-inches skillet pan, grease with oil and place it over medium heat.
2. Add onion, pepper and bacon, cook for 5 minutes or until slightly golden and then season with salt and black pepper.
3. Beat the eggs in a bowl, add ¼ cup of cheese and whisk until mixed.
4. When bacon is cooked, pour the egg mixture into the pan, spread evenly and cook for 5 minutes or until frittata is set.
5. In the meantime, switch on the broiler and let preheat.
6. When the frittata is set, sprinkle remaining cheese on the top, then place the pan under the broiler and cook until golden brown.
7. Let the frittata cool at room temperature, then cut it into four pieces, place each frittata piece in a heatproof glass meal prep container and store them in the refrigerator for 5 to 7 days.
8. When ready to serve, microwave frittata in their container for 1 to 2 minutes or until thoroughly heated.

Nutrition: Calories: 494 - **Fat:** 40g - **Protein**: 32g

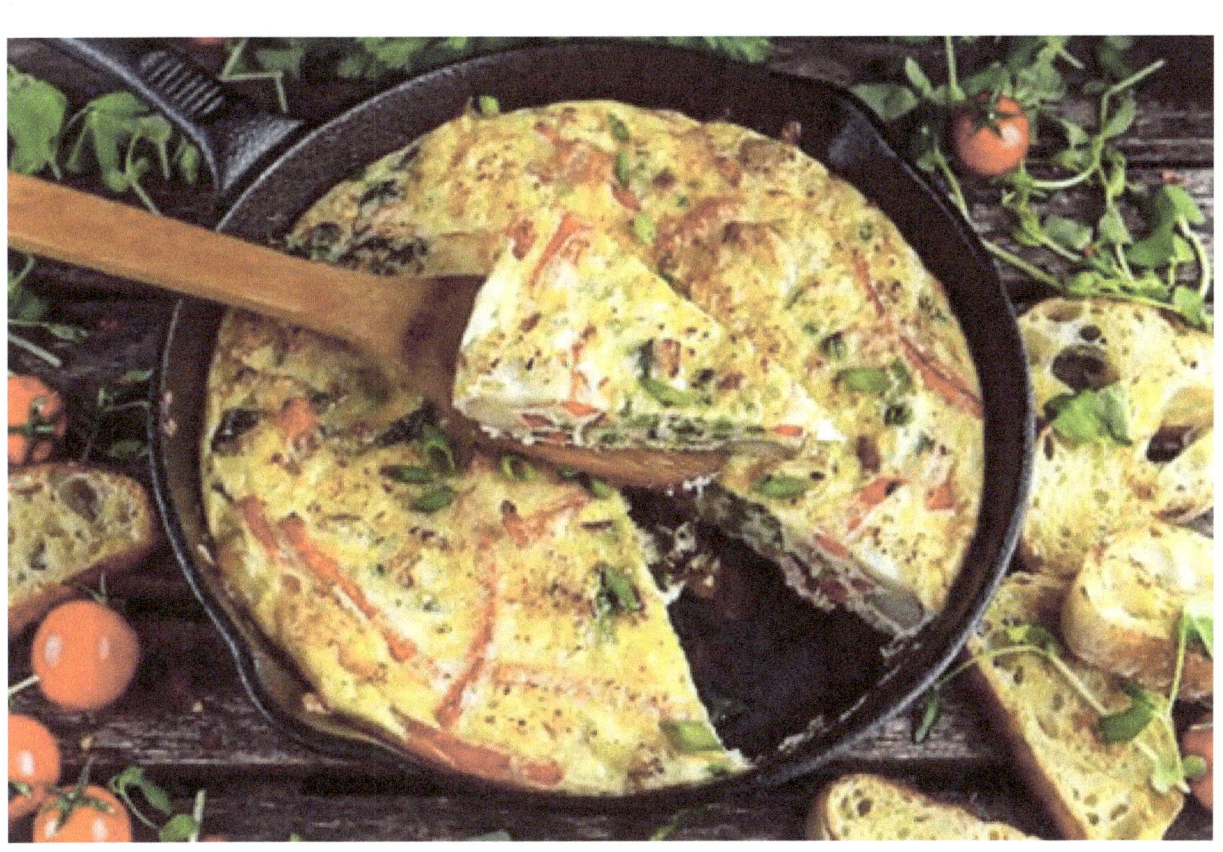

Pork Pie

Preparation time: 10 minutes **Cooking time:** 50 minutes **Servings:** 6

Ingredients:

- *crust:*
- 2 cups cracklings
- A pinch of salt
- ¼ cup flax meal
- 2 eggs
- 1 cup almond flour
- *filling:*
- 1 cup cheddar cheese, grated
- 4 eggs
- 12 ounces pork loin, chopped
- ½ cup cream cheese
- 1 red onion, chopped ¼ cup chives, chopped
- 6 bacon slices
- Salt and black pepper to the taste
- 2 garlic cloves, minced
- 2 tablespoons ghee

Directions:

1. In your food processor, mix cracklings with almond flour, flax meal, 2 eggs and salt and blend until you obtain a dough.
2. Transfer this to a pie pan and press well on the bottom.
3. Introduce in the oven at 350 degrees F and bake for 15 minutes.
4. Meanwhile, heat up a pan with the ghee over medium high heat, add garlic and onion, stir and cook for 5 minutes.
5. Add bacon, stir and cook for 5 minutes.
6. 6Add pork loin, cook until it's brown on all sides and take off heat.
7. In a bowl, mix eggs with salt, pepper, cheddar cheese and cream cheese and blend well.
8. Add chives and stir again.
9. Spread pork into pie pan, add eggs mix, introduce in the oven at 350 degrees F and bake for 25 minutes.
10. Leave the pie to cool down for a couple of minutes and serve.

Enjoy!

Nutrition: calories 455, fat 34, fiber 3, carbs 3, protein 33

Pate

Preparation time: 10 minutes **Cooking time:** 0 minutes **Servings:** 1

Ingredients:
- 3 radishes, thinly sliced Crusted
- bread slices for serving
- 4 ounces chicken livers, sautéed
- 3 tablespoons butter
- 1 teaspoon mixed thyme, sage and oregano, chopped
- Salt and black pepper to the taste

Directions:
1. In your food processor, mix chicken livers with thyme, sage, oregano, butter, salt and pepper and blend very well for a few minutes.
2. Spread on crusted bread slices and top with radishes slices.
3. Serve right away.

Enjoy!

Nutrition: calories 380, fat 40, fiber 5, carbs 1, protein 17

Zucchini Crusted Pizza

Preparation Time: 10 minutes **Cooking Time:** 45 minutes **Servings:** 6

Ingredients:
- 2 large eggs (beaten)
- 2 cups of zucchini (shredded, squeezed)
- ½ cup of mozzarella cheese (shredded)
- 1/3 cup of parmesan cheese (grated)
- ¼ cup of flour
- 1 tbsp. of olive oil
- 1 ½ tbsp. of basil (minced)
- 1 tsp. of thyme (minced)

For the toppings:
- 12 ounces of sweet red pepper (roasted, julienned)
- 1 cup of mozzarella cheese (shredded)
- ½ cup of turkey pepperoni (sliced)

Kitchen Equipment:
- oven
- pizza pan
- pizza cutter

Directions:
1. Preheat your oven at two hundred degrees Celsius.
2. Mix the first eight listed ingredients in a bowl.
3. Transfer the mixture to a greased pizza pan.
4. Spread the mixture and evenly press it to the base.
5. Bake for sixteen minutes.
6. Add the toppings on the pizza.
7. Bake for twelve minutes.
8. Slice the pizza using a pizza cutter.
9. Serve hot.

Nutrition:
- **Calories:** 226.3 - **Protein:** 13.6g - **Carbs:** 8.6g

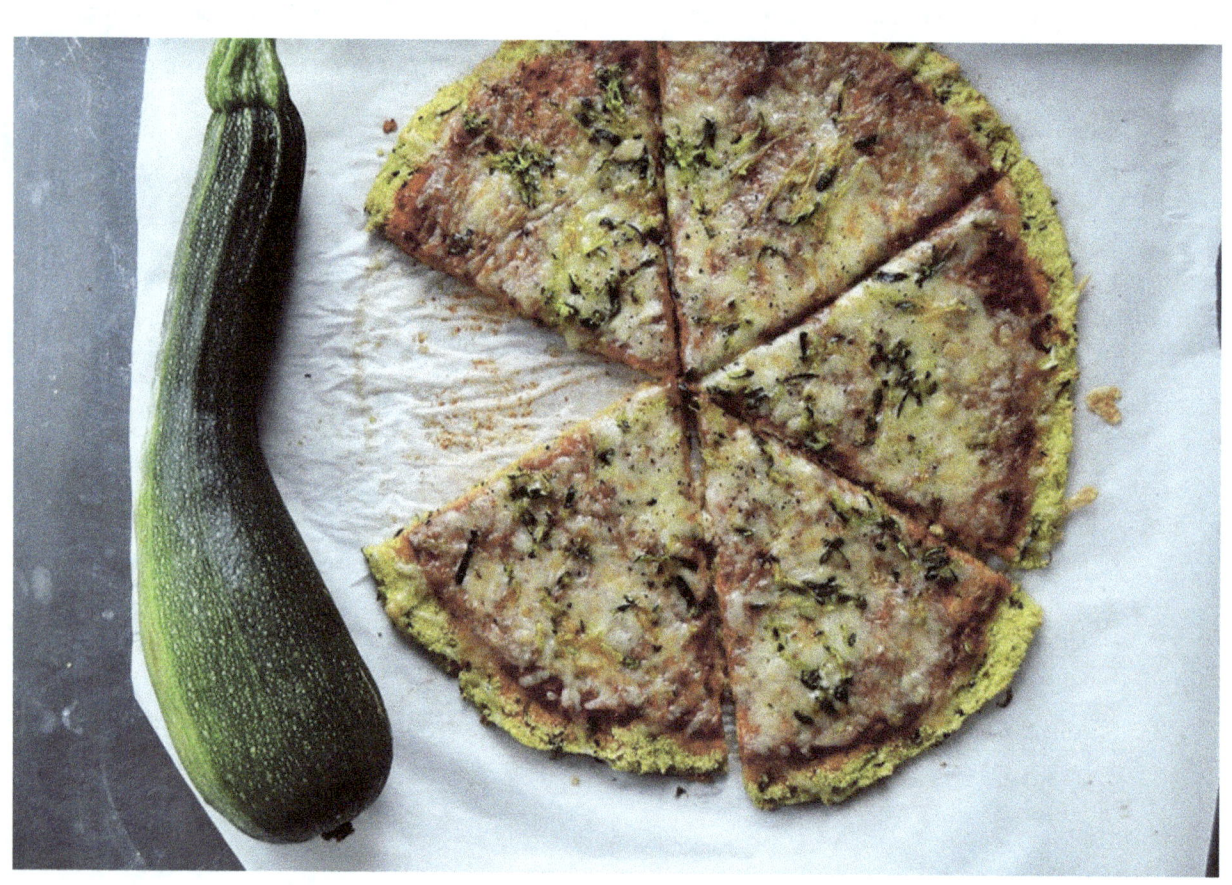

Noodles Soup

Preparation time: 10 minutes **Cooking time:** 15 minutes **Servings:** 8

Ingredients:
- 2 zucchinis, cut with a spiralizer
- ½ cup cilantro, chopped
- Lime wedges for serving
- 1 red bell pepper, sliced
- 2 tablespoons fish sauce
- 15 ounces canned coconut milk
- 1 pound chicken breasts, sliced
- 1 and ½ tablespoons curry paste
- 6 cups chicken stock
- 1 jalapeno pepper, chopped
- 1 tablespoon coconut oil
- 1 small yellow onion, chopped
- 2 garlic cloves, minced

Directions:
1. Heat up a pot with the oil over medium heat, add onion, stir and cook for 5 minutes.
2. Add garlic, jalapeno and curry paste, stir and cook for 1 minute.
3. Add stock and coconut milk, stir and bring to a boil.
4. Add red bell pepper, chicken and fish sauce, stir and simmer for
5. 4 minutes more.
6. Add cilantro, stir, cook for 1 minute and take off heat.
7. Divide zucchini noodles into soup bowls, add soup on top and serve with lime wedges on the side.

Enjoy!

Nutrition: calories 287, fat 14, fiber 2, carbs 7, protein 25

Roasted Cauliflower and Tahini Yogurt Sauce

Preparation Time: 10 minutes **Cooking Time:** 55 minutes **Servings:** 4

Ingredients:

- ¼ cup of parmesan cheese (grated)
- 3 tbsps. of olive oil
- 2 cloves of garlic (minced)
- ¼ tsp. of salt
- 1/3 tsp. of pepper
- 1 cauliflower (cut in four wedges)

For the sauce:

- ½ cup of Greek yogurt
- 1 tbsp. of lemon juice
- ½ tbsp. of tahini
- ¼ tsp. of salt
- 1 pinch of paprika
- Parsley (minced)

Kitchen Equipment:

- oven
- baking tray

Directions:

1. Preheat your oven at one hundred and fifty degrees Celsius.
2. Mix the first five ingredients.
3. Rub the mixture over the wedges of cauliflower.
4. Grease a baking tray with cooking spray.
5. Arrange the wedges of cauliflower on the baking tray.
6. Roast for forty minutes.
7. For the sauce, combine lemon juice, yogurt, seasonings, and tahini in a bowl.
8. Serve the cauliflower wedges and drizzle tahini sauce on top.

9. Garnish with parsley.

Nutrition: Calories: 179.6 **Protein:** 7.6g **Fat:** 15.4g

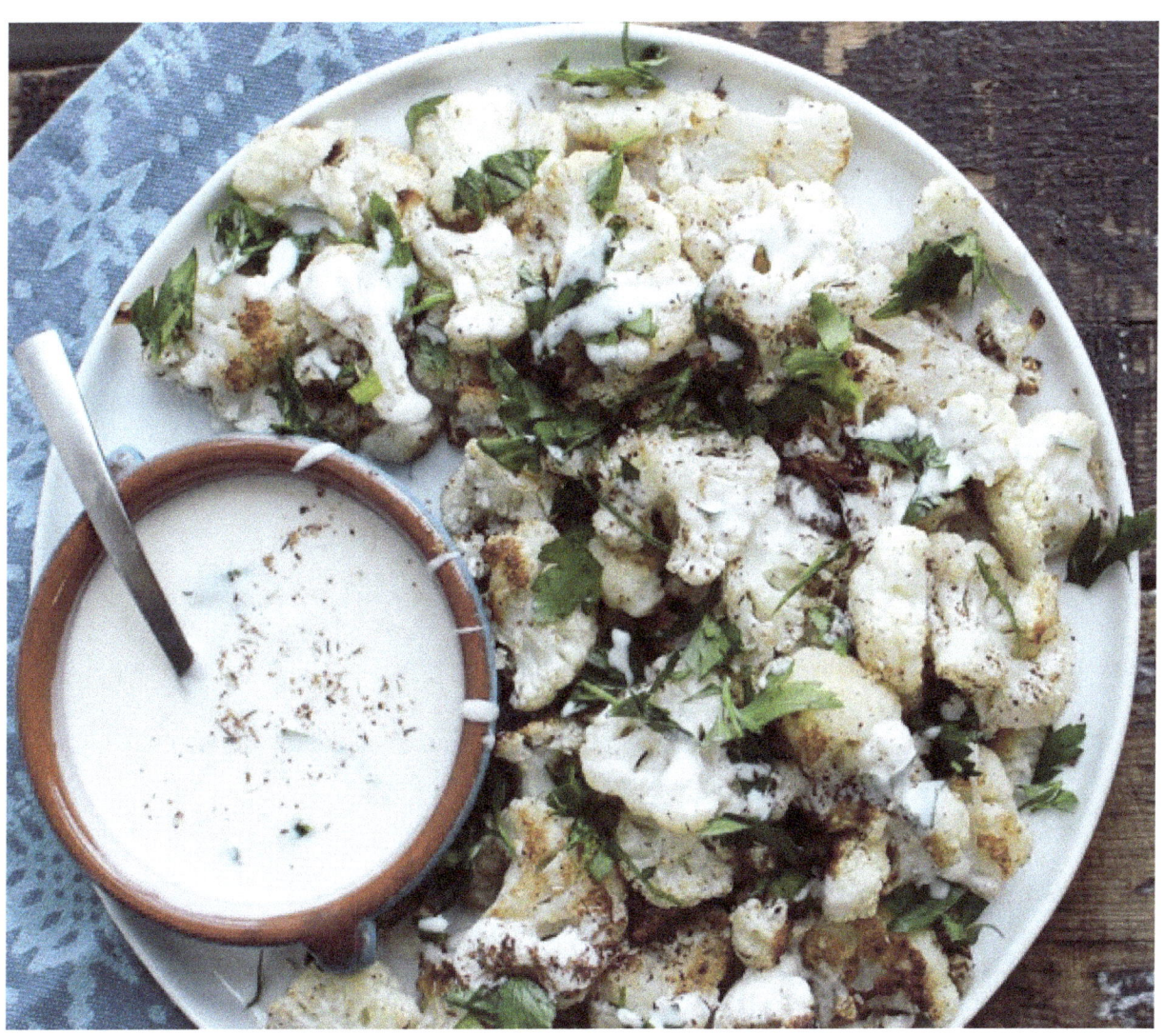

Spicy Tuna Kebab

Preparation Time: 4 minutes **Cooking Time:** 9 minutes **Servings:** 4

Ingredients:
- 4 tablespoon of Huy Fong chili garlic sauce
- 1 tablespoon of sesame oil infused with garlic
- 1 tablespoon of ginger, fresh, grated
- 1 tablespoon of garlic, minced
- 1 red onion, separated by petals
- 2 cups of bell peppers, red, green, yellow
- 1 can of whole water chestnuts
- ½ pound of fresh mushrooms halved
- 32 oz. of boneless tuna, chunks or steaks
- 1 Splenda packet
- 2 zucchinis, sliced
- 1 inch thick, keep skins on

Kitchen Equipment:
- blender
- zip-lock bag

Directions:

1. Layer the tuna spices and the oil and chili gravy, add the Splenda.
2. Quickly blend, either in a blender or by quickly whipping.
3. Brush onto the kabob pieces, make sure every piece is coated
4. Grill 4 minutes on each district, check to ensure the tuna is cooked to taste. Serving size is two skewers.
5. Mix the marinade ingredients and hide in a covered container in the fridge.
6. Place all the vegetables in one package in the fridge container in the fridge.

7. Place the tuna in a separate zip-lock bag.

Nutrition: Calories: 467 **Total Fat:** 18g **Protein:** 56g

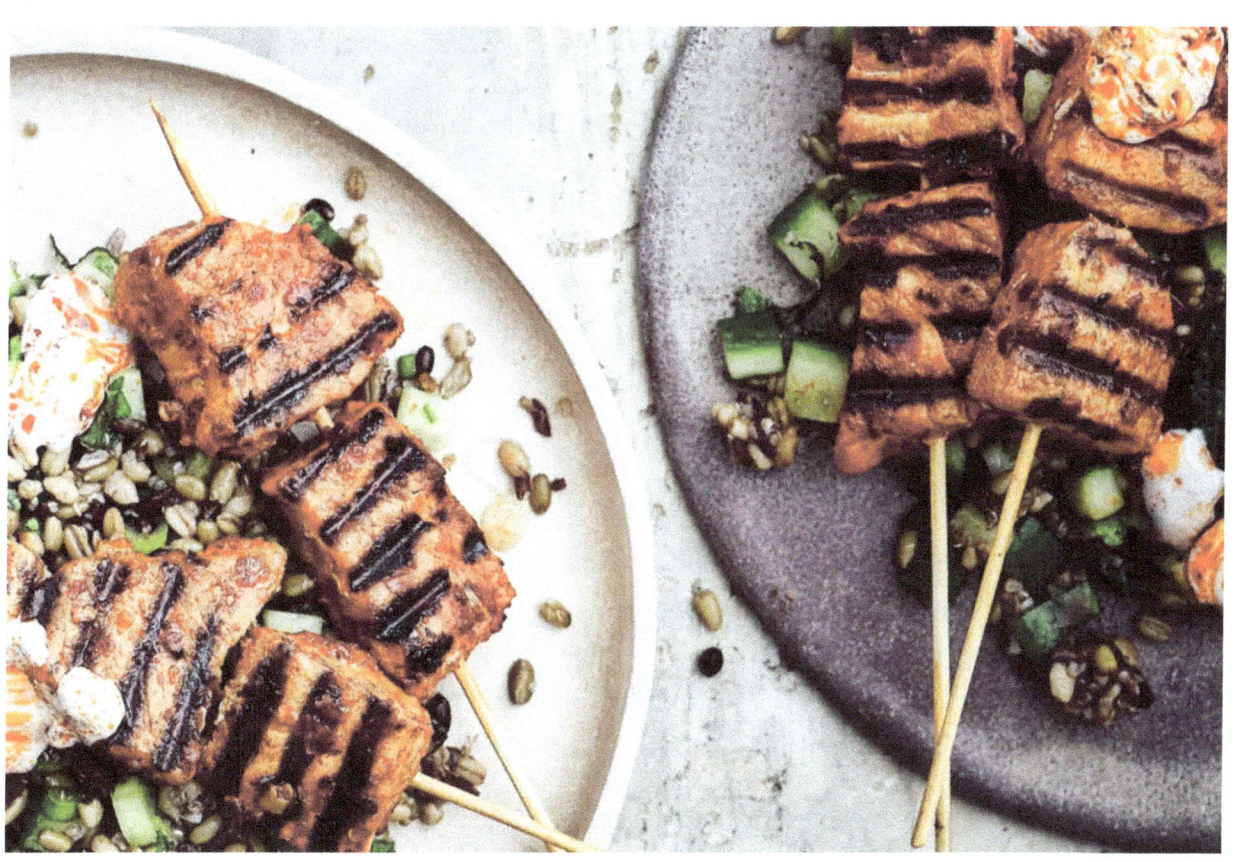

Asparagus Pries

Preparation Time: 10 minutes **Cooking Time:** 10 minutes **Servings:** 2

Ingredients:
- 10 medium organic asparagus spears
- 1 tbsp. of organic roasted red pepper, chopped
- ¼ cup of almond flour
- ½ tsp. of garlic powder
- ½ tsp. of smoked paprika
- 2 tbsp. of chopped parsley
- ½ cup of parmesan cheese, grated and full-fat
- 2 Organic eggs, beaten
- 3 tbsp. of mayonnaise, full-fat

Kitchen Equipment:
- oven
- food processor
- baking sheet

Directions:
1. Set the oven to 425 degrees and preheat.
2. Meanwhile, place cheese in a food processor, add garlic and parsley and pulse for 1 minute until fine mixture comes together.
3. Add almond flour, pulse for 30 seconds until just mixed, then tip the mixture into a bowl and season with paprika.
4. Break eggs into a shallow dish and whisk until beaten.
5. Working on one asparagus spear at a time, first dip into the egg mixture, then coat with the parmesan mixture and place it on a baking sheet.
6. Dip and coat more asparagus in the same manner, then arrange them on a baking sheet, 1-inch apart, and bake in the oven for 10 minutes or until asparagus is tender and nicely golden brown.

7. Meanwhile, place mayonnaise in a bowl, add red pepper and whisk until combined and chill the dip into the refrigerator until required.

8. Serve asparagus with prepared dip.

Nutrition: Calories: 453 **Fat:** 33.4g **Protein:** 19.1g

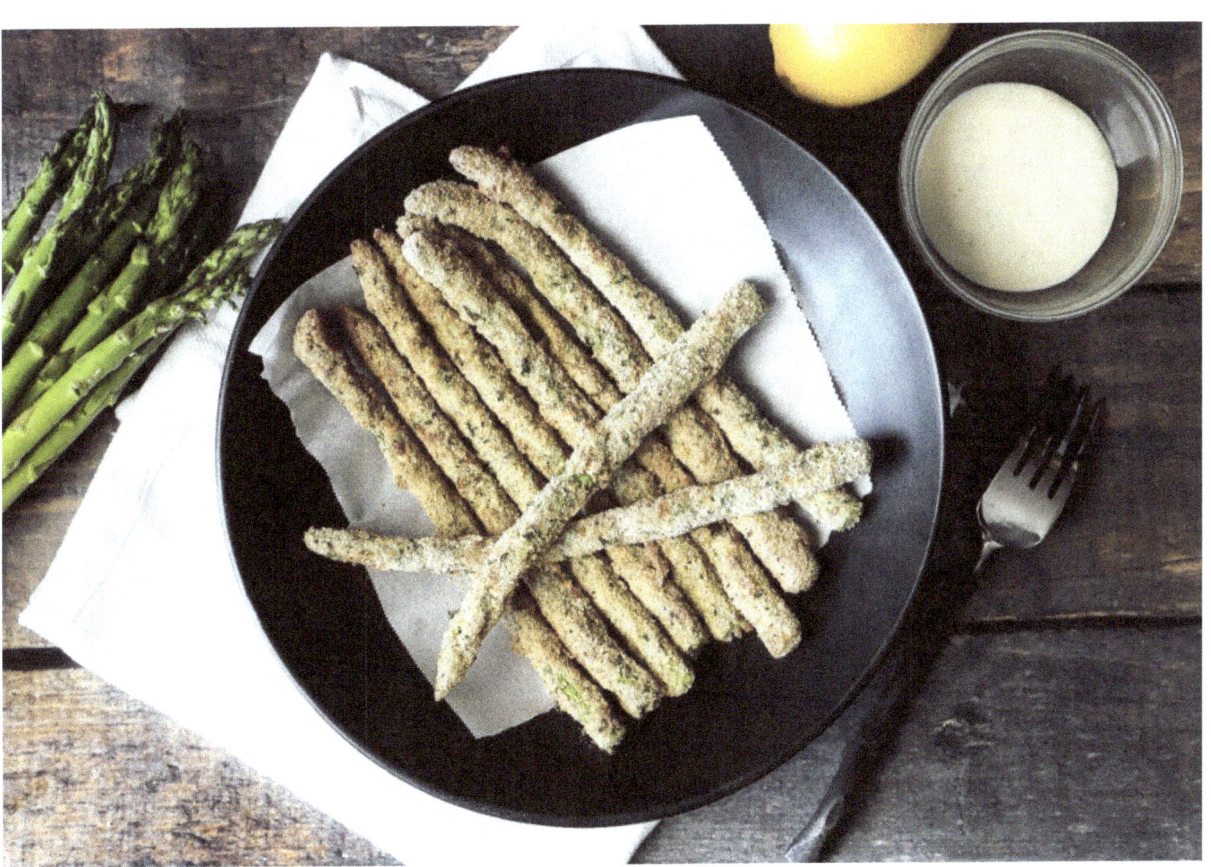

Garlicky green Beans

Gluten Free, Nut Free, Vegetarian

Preparation Time: 10 minutes **Cooking Time:** 10 minutes **Servings:** 4

Ingredients:
- 1-pound of green beans, stemmed
- 2 tablespoons of olive oil
- 1 teaspoon of minced garlic
- Sea salt
- Freshly ground black pepper
- ¼ cup of freshly grated Parmesan cheese

Kitchen Equipment:
- oven
- baking sheet
- aluminum foil
- large bowl

Directions:
1. Preheat the oven to 425°F.
2. Put aluminum foil in a baking sheet and set aside.
3. In a large bowl, toss together the green beans, olive oil, and garlic.
4. Season the beans lightly.
5. Arrange the beans on the baking sheet and roast them until they are tender and lightly browned, stirring them once, about 10 minutes.
6. Serve topped with the Parmesan cheese.

Nutrition: Calories: 104 - **Fat:** 9g - **Protein:** 4g

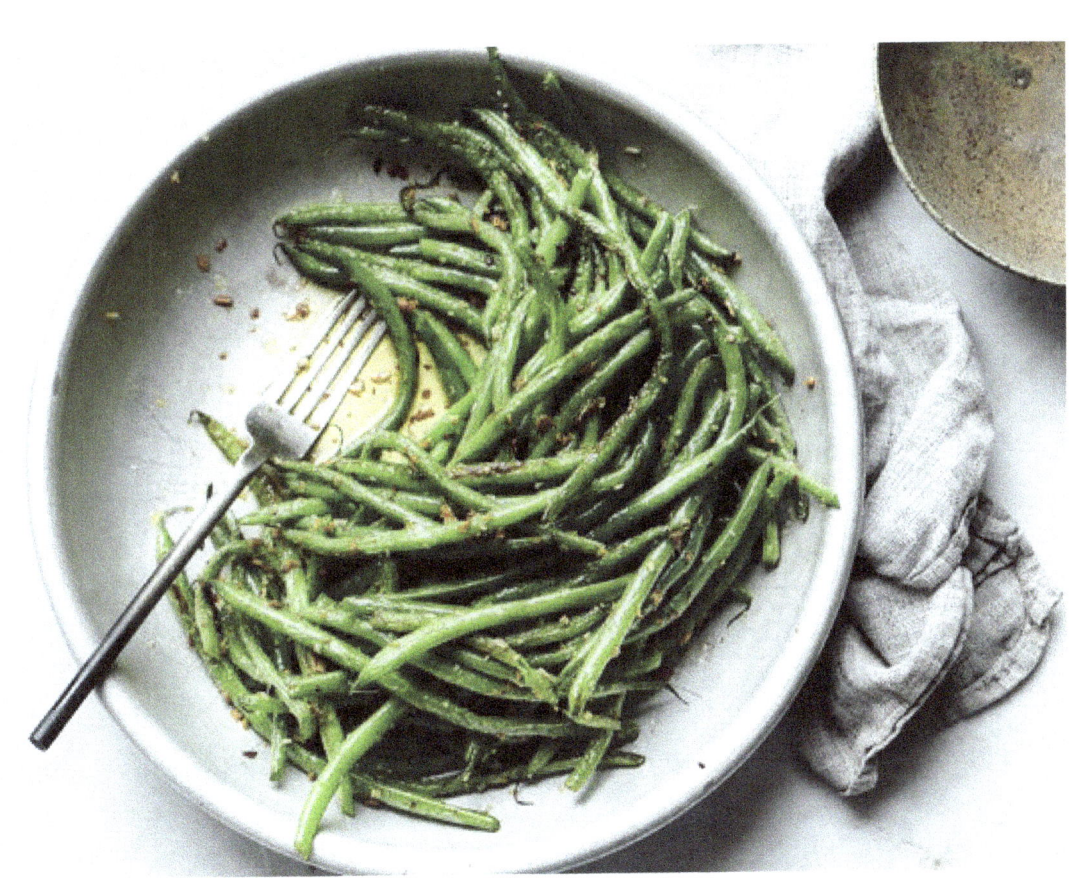

Creamy Chicken Pot Pie Soup

Preparation Time: 20 minutes **Cooking Time:** 35 minutes **Servings:** 6

Ingredients:

- 2 tablespoons of extra-virgin olive oil (divided)
- 1 pound (454 g) of skinless chicken breast (cut into ½-inch chunks)
- 1 cup of mushrooms (quartered)
- 2 celery stalks (chopped)
- 1 onion (chopped)
- 1 tablespoon of garlic (minced)
- 5 cups of low-sodium chicken broth
- 1 cup of green beans (chopped)
- ¼ cup of cream cheese
- 1 cup of heavy whipping cream
- 1 tablespoon of fresh thyme (chopped)
- Salt and black pepper (to taste)

Kitchen Equipment:

- stockpot

Directions:

1. Cook the olive oil in a stockpot over medium-high heat until shimmering.
2. Add the chicken chunks to the pot and sauté for 10 minutes or until well browned.
3. Transfer the chicken to a plate. Set aside until ready to use.
4. Cook the remaining olive oil in the stockpot over medium-high heat.
5. Add the mushrooms, celery, onion, and garlic to the pot and sauté for 6 minutes or until fork-tender.
6. Pour the chicken broth over, then add the cooked chicken chunks to the pot.

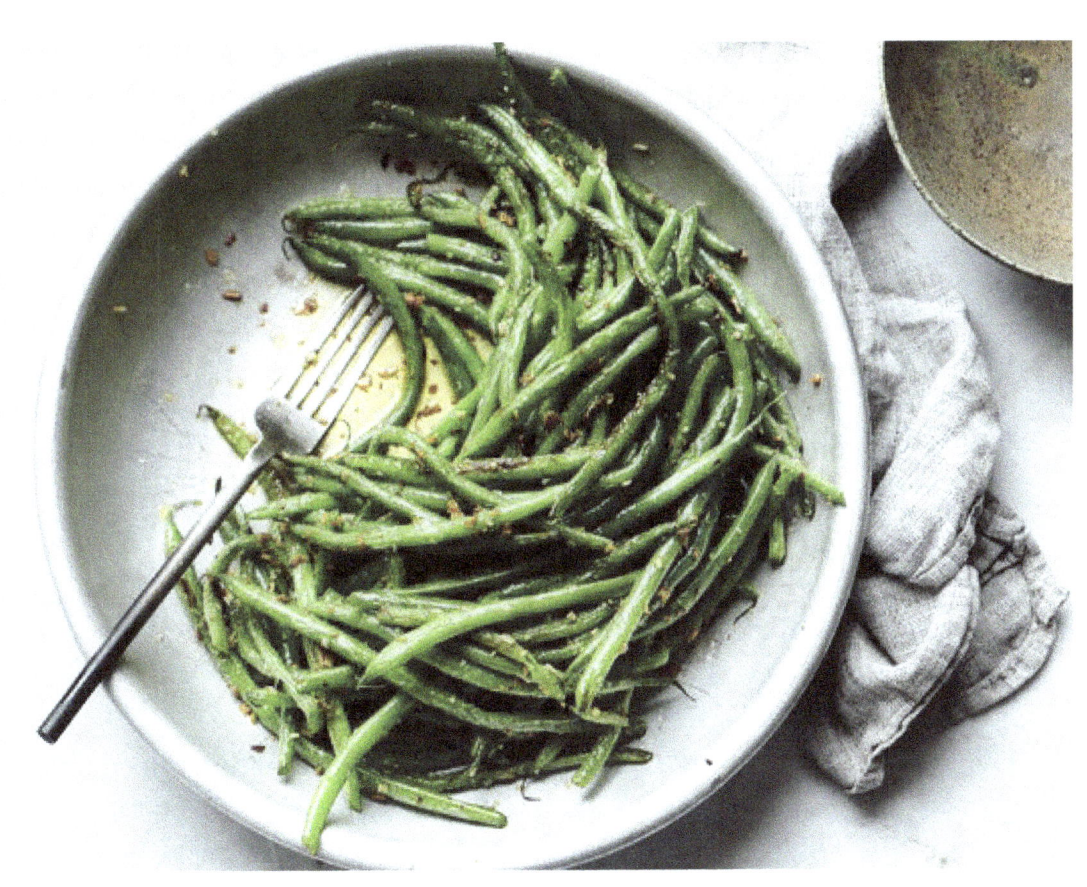

Creamy Chicken Pot Pie Soup

Preparation Time: 20 minutes **Cooking Time:** 35 minutes **Servings:** 6

Ingredients:

- 2 tablespoons of extra-virgin olive oil (divided)
- 1 pound (454 g) of skinless chicken breast (cut into ½-inch chunks)
- 1 cup of mushrooms (quartered)
- 2 celery stalks (chopped)
- 1 onion (chopped)
- 1 tablespoon of garlic (minced)
- 5 cups of low-sodium chicken broth
- 1 cup of green beans (chopped)
- ¼ cup of cream cheese
- 1 cup of heavy whipping cream
- 1 tablespoon of fresh thyme (chopped)
- Salt and black pepper (to taste)

Kitchen Equipment:

- stockpot

Directions:

1. Cook the olive oil in a stockpot over medium-high heat until shimmering.//
2. Add the chicken chunks to the pot and sauté for 10 minutes or until well browned.
3. Transfer the chicken to a plate. Set aside until ready to use.
4. Cook the remaining olive oil in the stockpot over medium-high heat.
5. Add the mushrooms, celery, onion, and garlic to the pot and sauté for 6 minutes or until fork-tender.
6. Pour the chicken broth over, then add the cooked chicken chunks to the pot.

7. Stir to mix well, and bring the soup to a boil.

8. Set heat to low, and simmer for 15 minutes or until the vegetables are soft and the internal temperature of the chicken reaches at least 165ºF (74ºC).

9. Mix in the green beans, cream cheese, cream, thyme, salt, and black pepper, then simmer for 3 minutes more.

10. Remove the soup from the stockpot and serve hot.

Nutrition: Calories: 338 **Total fat:** 26.1g **Fiber:** 2.2g

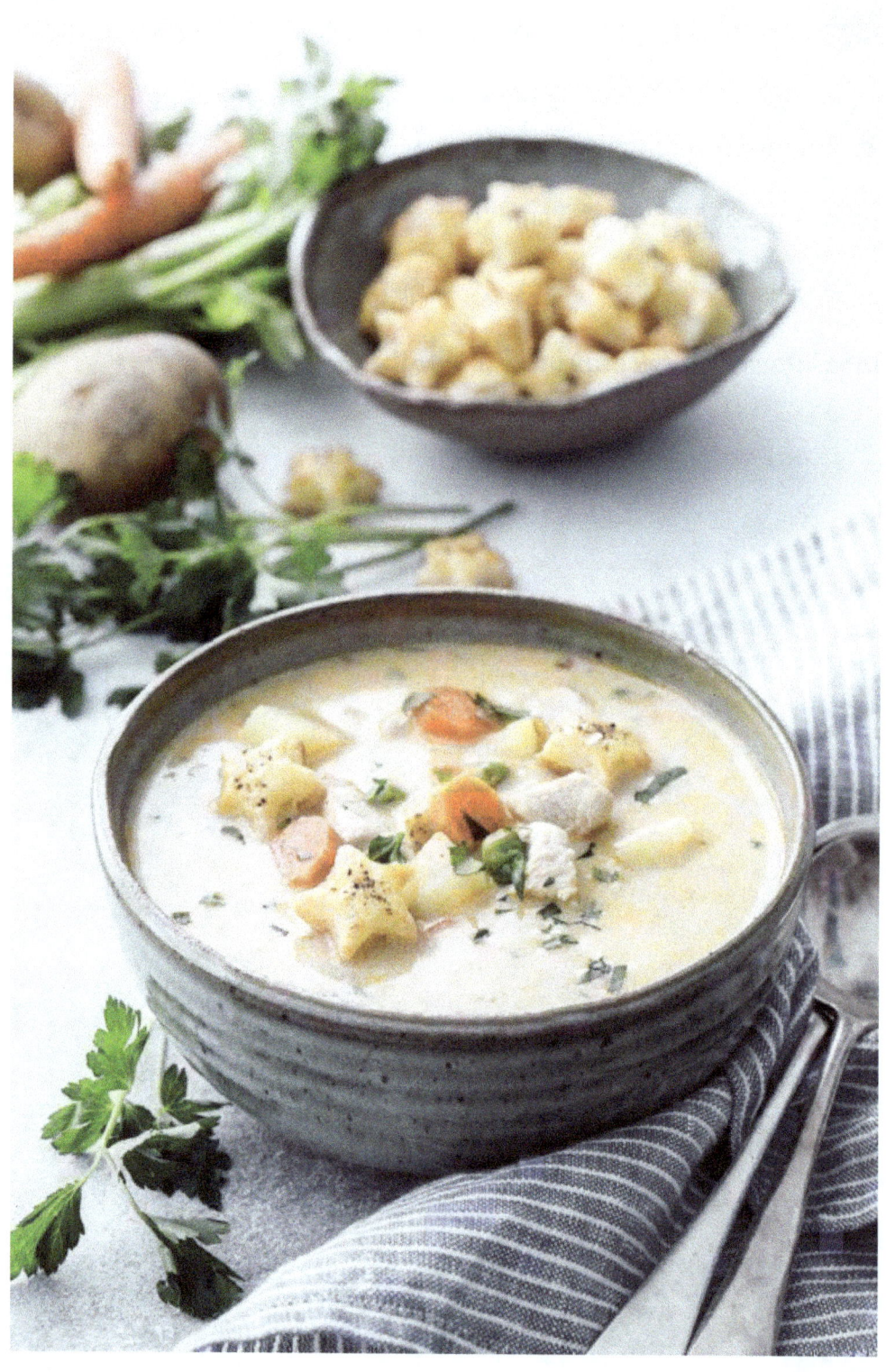

www.ingramcontent.com/pod-product-compliance
Lightning Source LLC
Chambersburg PA
CBHW081508080526
44589CB00017B/2687